Ethics and Law in Dental Hygiene

SECOND EDITION

Phyllis L. Beemsterboer, RDH, EdD

Associate Dean for Academic Affairs
School of Dentistry
Oregon Health & Science University
Portland, Oregon

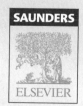

SAUNDERS

ELSEVIER

SAUNDERS
ELSEVIER

11830 Westline Industrial Drive
St. Louis, Missouri 63146

Notice

Neither the Publisher nor the Author assumes any responsibility for any loss or injury and/or damage to persons or property arising out of or related to any use of the material contained in this book. It is the responsibility of the treating practitioner, relying on independent expertise and knowledge of the patient, to determine the best treatment and method of application for the patient.

The Publisher

Library of Congress Cataloging-in-Publication Data
Beemsterboer, Phyllis.
   Ethics and law in dental hygiene / Phyllis L. Beemsterboer.—2nd ed.
     p. ; cm.
   Includes bibliographical references and index.
   ISBN 978-1-4160-6235-6 (pbk. : alk. paper)
   1. Dental hygienists—Legal status, laws, etc.—United States. 2. Dental ethics—United States. I. Title.
   [DNLM: 1. Dental Hygienists—ethics—United States. 2. Dental Hygienists—legislation & jurisprudence—United States. 3. Ethics, Dental—United States. WU 33 AA1 B414e 2010]
   KF2910.D3B44 2010
   344.7304'13—dc22

          2008054145

Vice President and Publisher: Linda Duncan
Senior Editor: John Dolan
Managing Editor: Kristin Hebberd
Associate Developmental Editor: Joslyn Dumas
Publishing Services Manager: Hemamalini Rajendrababu
Project Manager: Shereen Jameel
Design: Teresa McBryan

Printed in the United States of America

Last digit is the print number: 9   8   7   6   5

Working together to grow libraries in developing countries

www.elsevier.com | www.bookaid.org | www.sabre.org

ELSEVIER   BOOK AID International   Sabre Foundation

Contributors

Gail L. Aamodt, RDH, MS
Assistant Professor Dental Hygiene Program
Clinical Education Coordinator
School of Dental Health Science
Pacific University
Hillsboro, Oregon

Karen Adams, MD
Clinical Consultant
Center for Ethics in Health Care
OB/GYN Residency Program Director
Oregon Health & Science University
Portland, Oregon

Kathleen H. Alvarez, RDH, MS
Assistant Professor
Department of Dental Hygiene, Cypress College
Adjunct Instructor
Department of Dental Hygiene, West Los Angeles College
Cypress, California

Kathryn Ann Atchison, DDS, MPH
Vice Provost and Dean
Intellectual Property and Industry Relations
University of California at Los Angeles
Los Angeles, California

Cheryl A. Cameron, RDH, PhD, JD
Vice Provost for Academic Personnel
Office of the Provost
Professor
Dental Public Health Sciences
School of Dentistry
University of Washington
Seattle, Washington

Michelle Carr, RDH, MA
Associate Professor and Director
Dental Hygiene—Section of Primary Care
College of Dentistry
The Ohio State University
Columbus, Ohio

Frank Catalanotto, DMD
Professor
Department of Public Health
University of Florida
Gainesville, Florida

Gary Chiodo, DMD, PhD
Chief Integrity Officer
Center for Ethics in Health Care
Oregon Health & Science University
Portland, Oregon

Christina B. DeBiase, EdD
Associate Dean
Administration Dentistry
West Virginia University
Morgantown, West Virginia

Debra L. Gerger, RDH, MPH
Department Chair
Department of Dental Hygiene
West Coast University
Anaheim, California

Marcia A. Gladwin, EdD
Director
Dental Hygiene Program
School of Dentistry
West Virginia University
Morgantown, West Virginia

Kim L. Halula, PhD
Associate Dean College of Health Sciences
Interim Chair Physician Assistant Studies
Marquette University
Milwaukee, Wisconsin

Thomas K. Hasegawa, DDS
Professor
Director of Clinical Services
Baylor College of Dentistry
Texas A&M University
Dallas, Texas

Anne High, RDH, MS
Instructor
Department of Dental Hygiene
Rochester Community and Technical College
Rochester, Minnesota

Stephanie Bossenberger James, RDH, MS
Professor
Department of Dental Hygiene
Weber State University
Ogden, Utah

Donna Lesser, RDH, BS
Director
Dental Hygiene Program
Riverside Community College
Moreno Valley, California

Carla Loiacono, RDH, MS
Director of Dental Hygiene
Institute of Medical Education
San Jose, California

Phyllis Martina, BSDH, MBA
School Manager
School and Institutional Sales
Hu-Friedy Manufacturing Company, Inc.
Chicago, Illinois

Ann Louise McCann, PhD
Director of Planning and Assessment
Baylor College of Dentistry
Department of Academic Affairs
Texas A&M Health Science Center
Dallas, Texas

Patricia J. Nunn RDH, MS
Director Emeritus, Dean of Students
Associate Director of Education
Utah College of Dental Hygiene
Orem, Utah

John Odom, PhD
Associate Professor (Retired)
Department of Primary Care
College of Dentistry
The Ohio State University
Columbus, Ohio

Pamela Overman, BS, MS, EdD
Professor and Associate Dean for Academic Affairs
School of Dentistry
University of Missouri–Kansas City
Kansas City, Missouri

David Ozar, PhD
Professor
Center for Ethics and Social Justice
Loyola University Lake Shore Campus
Professor
Philosophy Department
Loyola University
Water Tower Campus
Chicago, Illinois

Alvin B. Rosenblum, DDS
Professor
School of Dentistry
University of Southern California
Los Angeles, California

Catherine Salveson, RN, PhD
Associate Professor
School of Nursing
Oregon Health & Science University
Portland, Oregon

Michelle M. Singley, RDH, EdM
Dental Hygiene Coordinator
Lewis and Clark Community College
Godfrey, Illinois

Mary Turner, RDH, MS
Dean
Division of Science and Allied Health
Sacramento City College
Sacramento, California

Donna Wittmayer, RDH, BS, MS
Director
Department of Dental Hygiene
Clark College
Vancouver, Washington

Pamela Zarkowski, JD, MPH, BSDH
Executive Associate Dean and Professor
Department of Patient Management
School of Dentistry
University of Detroit Mercy
Detroit, Michigan

This book is dedicated to my husband,
Joseph R. Jedrychowski,

and

the Beemsterboer/Jedrychowski families
who mean everything to me.

PLB

Preface

Dental hygiene as a profession is well-positioned to continue its growth, as it has since its beginnings in the early part of the twentieth century. Dental hygiene students no longer have to rely on one textbook to provide all the materials and references from which to study and learn. Now, numerous textbooks, on a wide variety of subject content, are available to dental hygiene educators and students. The subject of ethics and law has always been included in comprehensive dental hygiene textbook volumes. However, the complexity of the modern world and the impact of technology and science on the health care professions have increased the challenge of providing ethical care in the daily functioning of the dental hygienist. Ethics and law now require a separate title that addresses the subject in the proper scope and depth for the dental hygiene student. *Ethics and Law in Dental Hygiene* meets this need in both the educational and professional markets, serving as a valuable tool for new and practicing dental hygienists.

Background and Importance to the Profession

Dental ethics as an area of study came into its own in the 1980s as the result of the efforts of a group of scholars at Georgetown University in Washington, D.C. From this small visionary group came an ethics study network organization, several workshop and consensus activities, and ultimately three dental ethics textbooks. All three textbooks addressed the role of the dental hygienist in some way in the provision of dental health care to the public. An increased emphasis on and awareness of ethics in the various dental professions has given way to more specialized titles and to groups that work toward increasing the social responsibility and ethical conduct of oral health care professionals. The importance of ethics is also evidenced by the many dental hygiene educators who are active in the American Society for Dental Ethics (ASDE), an association of educators, philosophers, and practitioners who are dedicated to the ongoing study of ethical issues and education with the goal of promoting professional responsibility and conduct for the public we serve. The second edition of *Ethics and Law in Dental Hygiene* provides the most up-to-date ethics coverage for dental hygiene students and practitioners.

Audience

This text is devoted to the topic of ethics and law for the dental hygienist, a professional who holds a unique place in the provision of oral health care services. The book provides information and guidance for entry-level dental hygiene students as well as experienced practitioners looking to continue their professional development.

Organization

This textbook is organized into three sections, with the first two sections focusing on content and the third devoted to application. The first section presents the foundational aspects of ethics and introduces an ethical decision-making tool for the analysis of ethical dilemmas. Legal concepts are discussed in the second section and provide information on state practice acts and risk management.

The third section provides 25 case scenarios authored by various contributors with expertise in dental and dental hygiene ethics for the reader to discuss and analyze. Questions to stimulate thought and discussion are included as well, and the ethical decision-making model can be applied to each of the cases. Although hypothetical cases, the situations presented are a culmination of many years of experience in dentistry and dental hygiene and provide a variety of material for lively and fruitful discussion sessions. Four "testlets" are also included to help prepare students for the National Board Dental Hygiene Examination (NBDHE). A testlet is a short clinical scenario with a series of associated test items that focus on critical thinking and problem-solving skills. Lastly, a listing of suggested activities and projects helps expand upon the topics presented in the textbook and encourages additional thought and discussion.

Key Features

- Coverage of ethics and law is balanced equally throughout and presented in a clear and concise manner to demystify these often complex topics.
- Concepts are discussed in the context of real-world relevance to help readers apply the knowledge to everyday situations.

- A six-step decision-making model equips readers with a framework to tackle ethical situations.
- Contributors include educators and practitioners who are renowned leaders in the ethics of dentistry and dental hygiene.
- A wealth of case studies and additional activities cover a wide range of situations and provide readers with opportunities to hone their ability to make sound ethical and legal decisions.
- Chapter key terms and a back-of-book glossary help ensure content mastery of the unique and often challenging language used within law and ethics.

New to this Edition

- A new chapter, "Social Responsibility and Justice," addresses timely issues such as access to oral health care and health disparities.
- Returning chapters are fully revised and expanded, including coverage of key topics such as the Health Insurance Portability and Accountability Act (HIPAA).
- Additional case scenarios written by experts within dental and dental hygiene ethics provide for discussion, analysis, and application.
- "Testlets" encourage critical thinking, challenge problem-solving skills, and help prepare students for the case-based National Board Dental Hygiene Examination (NBDHE) by using the same format.
- The newly revised editions of the American Dental Hygiene Association (ADHA) and American Dental Association (ADA) codes of ethics are provided in full as appendices.

Wherever you are in your dental hygiene career, *Ethics and Law in Dental Hygiene* is an excellent foundation and a valuable reference to guide you through this complex subject matter with ease and understanding.

Phyllis L. Beemsterboer

Acknowledgments

The collaborators for this edition are educators who are devoted to the education of dental hygienists. My deepest appreciation goes to Cheryl Cameron and Pam Zarkowski, dental hygiene educators and administrators who also are attorneys. Bioethics experts David Ozar and Frank Catalanotto were most generous with their time and expertise.

I am grateful to my colleagues at the Center for Health Care Ethics at Oregon Health & Science University and those from the American Society for Dental Ethics. They continue to counsel, teach, and inspire me.

Phyllis L. Beemsterboer

Contents

8 Dental Hygienist–Patient Relationship, 119

CHERYL A. CAMERON AND PAMELA ZARKOWSKI

9 Dental Hygienist–Dentist-Employer Relationship, 139

CHERYL A. CAMERON AND PAMELA ZARKOWSKI

SECTION **III**

SIMULATIONS AND APPLICATIONS

Case Studies, Testlets, and Activities, 169

SECTION I

ETHICS

CHAPTER 1

Ethics and Professionalism

PHYLLIS L. BEEMSTERBOER

LEARNING OUTCOMES

- Describe the role of the dental hygienist in health care.
- Explain the relationship between the health care provider and the patient.
- Describe the aspects of a true profession as they apply to dentistry and dental hygiene.
- Discuss the theory of competency and skill acquisition for the dental hygienist.
- Compare educational competencies and practice standards.
- Identify the traits of a professional dental hygienist.

KEY TERMS

accreditation

competency

duty

licensure

oath

peer review

professional traits

professionalism

standards

traits

value

From its inception in the early 1900s, the profession of dental hygiene has been concerned with the public good and with advocating methods of preserving oral health. The first *oath* written for dental hygienists called upon Apollo, the god of health, and Hygeia, the goddess of health, to help each practitioner in performing the "sacred duty of teaching to the public, particularly children and young people, by precept, lecture and every other available mode of instruction, the value of dental health as a priceless possession."[1,3]

The dentists who pioneered this special field of endeavor positioned the dental hygienist as the oral preventive therapist because of their vision of the day when dental disease could be prevented by following a system of treatment and cleanliness.

The original intent of the first oath was preserved in a revised and modernized version adopted by the Board of Trustees of the American Dental Hygienists' Association (ADHA) in 1979 and is still in use today. This oath, which is affirmed by numerous dental hygiene students before or at the time of graduation from their formal education and training program, captures the essence of the public mission of the profession. The following, reprinted from Steele,[1] recalls that original oath, which has been updated since by the ADHA (www.adha.org/aboutadha/dhoath.htm):

> In my practice as a dental hygienist,
> I affirm my personal and professional commitment
> To improve the oral health of the public,
> To advance the art and science of dental hygiene,
> And to promote high standards of quality care.
> I pledge continually to improve my professional
> Knowledge and skills, to render a full measure
> Of service to each patient entrusted to my care,
> And to uphold the highest standards of professional
> Competence and personal conduct in the interest
> Of the dental hygiene profession and the public it serves.

Over the years, the profession of dental hygiene has evolved and changed with requirements for formalized education, regulation by licensure, and increased scope of practice. In addition, the public served by all health care providers has changed with the advent of new diseases, the development of advanced treatment methods, and a continually increasing human life span. However, dental hygiene retains its original focus on the public good, as well as its primary role in the prevention of dental disease and promotion of oral health.

Society recognizes that health care providers, by virtue of their education and special skills, are appropriately held to a higher standard than can be expressed exclusively by legislative mandate. Thus these higher standards are expressed in professional codes of ethics and are enforced by those within the profession. This is called *self-regulating* or *self-policing behavior* and represents an increased level of trust on the part of the public. In essence, the public agrees that it is neither qualified nor in a position to evaluate the adequacy of treatment provided by health care professionals. Therefore the public trusts these professions to perform their own evaluations. Ethical dental hygienists willingly accept the **duty** of self-regulation, both in judging their colleagues and in submitting to **peer review,** to ensure quality care for the public.

*E*thics is about character and courage and how we meet the challenge when doing the right thing will cost more than we want to pay.

JOSEPHSON INSTITUTE

■ The Health Care Provider

All health care providers are granted special rights and responsibilities when they choose and enter a career in the biomedical fields. In the past, becoming a professional in medicine, dentistry, or the allied disciplines was considered a calling. Once specialized training was completed, the individual became a member of a profession, defined as a limited group of persons who have acquired some special skill and are therefore able to perform that function in society better than the average person (Box 1-1).[3] In the corporate

---

BOX 1-1

Characteristics of a True Profession

- Specialized body of knowledge of value to society
- Intensive academic course of study
- Standards of practice
- External recognition by society
- Code of ethics
- Organized association
- Service orientation

Data from Motlley WE: Ethics, jurisprudence and history for the dental hygienist, *ed 3, Philadelphia, 1983, Lea & Febiger.*

world, success is measured by financial gain. For the health care professional, the patient's welfare is placed above profit. Because of this ideal, society has granted the health care professional a certain status that carries prestige, power, and the right to apply special knowledge and skill.

When patients seek care from any health care provider, they expect to receive the best care from a professional and ethical practitioner. The health care services provided involve technical skill, appropriate knowledge, critical judgment and, most importantly, caring. Patients perceive this essence of caring and respond to it. In the delivery of health care, trust is the critical foundation for the relationship that develops between the person seeking services—the patient or client—and the health care provider—the professional. The patient is aware that the health care provider has certain knowledge and skills; the graduation certificate and state license hanging on the wall are proof of that fact. However, the caring that the patient seeks gives the provider of dental hygiene services the greatest opportunity for professional service and satisfaction. An understanding of ethical issues and an awareness of the ethical obligations inherent in the provision of health care enable the dental hygienist to deal effectively with the problems of patients and their communities.

The importance and need for professionalism in all areas of health care have been extensively discussed and written about. Educators in medicine, dentistry, and dental hygiene have shared the importance of fostering professionalism and the fact that students must be immersed in clinical learning environments that model the highest principles.[4]

A number of medical organizations have focused on how to reemphasize the essence of professionalism in health care. The Institute of Medicine has produced several reports on this topic, and a project by a consortium of internal medicine groups led to the publication "Medical Professionalism in the New Millennium: A Physician Charter."[5] The authors advocated that everyone "involved in health care" use the charter to engage in discussions to strengthen the ethical underpinning of professional relationships. The Physician Charter sets out three fundamental principles that are not new but reinforce the foundation of the medical profession as one of service to others. The ethical principles of the primacy of patient welfare (beneficence and nonmaleficence) and patient autonomy are listed first; the principle of social justice is the third main tenet. The desired goal was to reinvigorate the value of professionalism that includes social responsibility: the ethic of care, and access to that care, for all members of society.

Professionalism is rooted in a relationship or contract with society. Ministry, medicine, and law grew from medieval guilds that were established in universities centuries ago. Entrance into these fields was controlled through the awarding of educational credentials. Early dental practitioners were itinerant barbers, and the road to professional status moved from apprenticeship to education through the establishment of professional schools.[6] Developing an educational process gave the members control over entry into the occupation and the size of the labor force. Because of their smaller number and their education, professionals became trustees of the community and took leadership positions in their societies.[7] This led to the public understanding that the professional person's knowledge is linked with service in the interest of the local community. Ultimately, the professional came to be defined as someone learned, publicly licensed, and supported by a collegial organization of peers committed to an ethic of service to clients and the public.[8] The professions then are much like universities and college in this sense—given a unique charter that grants autonomy and special status for a public purpose.

■ The Dental Hygienist

The dental hygienist is a professional oral health care provider—an individual who has completed a required higher education accredited program; demonstrated knowledge, skills, and behaviors required by the college or university for graduation; passed a written national board examination; and successfully performed certain clinical skills on a state or regional examination. Because of these accomplishments, the state then grants this individual a license to practice the profession for which he or she completed training and education. By taking this step, the state is assuring the public that this licensed individual is competent to practice. That is the reason that a board of dentistry or a dental practice act exists: to protect the public's health and safety.

A dental hygienist provides educational, clinical, and therapeutic services supporting the total health of the patient through the promotion of optimal oral health. Because of these functions, the dental hygienist has been defined as a preventive oral health care professional.

*A*n investment in knowledge always pays the best interest.

BENJAMIN FRANKLIN

To be considered a profession, a specific field or area of study traditionally must have several characteristics. These include a specialized body of knowledge and skill of value to society, an intensive academic course of study, set standards of practice determined and regulated by the group, external recognition by society, a code of ethics, an organized association, and a service ethic. What separates the professional from the layperson is this specialized knowledge, which is exclusive to the professional group. Because being a professional is considered desirable, many careers and occupations aspire to this level. Real estate agents, auto mechanics, and culinary chefs all use the term *professional* to indicate a desired level of competency and quality performance. However, the true professions are still considered to be medicine, dentistry, ministry, and law because they possess all the characteristics previously listed.

Moreover, a profession incurs an obligation by virtue of its relationship with society—something that is affirmed and reaffirmed over time. When an individual enters a course of professional study, learning about the tenets of the profession and its inherent obligations is part of the educational program. The Hippocratic Oath, dentist's pledge, and the dental hygiene oath are examples of outward signs that reflect acceptance of the professional obligation. Professionalism is demonstrated through a foundation of clinical competence, communication skills, and ethical and legal understanding, upon which is built the aspiration to and wise application of the principles of professionalism. These principles are excellence, humanism, accountability, and altruism.[9]

▪ Professionalism

The expectations of the public regarding health care have changed and evolved over the years. People have become increasingly knowledgeable, involved, and active in their own health care decisions. This change evolved from a traditional relationship between the practitioner and the patient. Ozar[10] described this evolution in his classic article in which he developed the three models of *professionalism:* the commercial model, the guild model, and the interactive model. These models are not intended to reflect how dental care has been delivered in the past but provide an examination of how the obligations of provider and patient should be established from a moral perspective.

Commercial Model

The commercial model describes a relationship in which dentistry is a commodity, a simple selling and buying of services. The patient is the consumer and the dentist is the producer. The dental needs of the patient are not as important as what the patient is willing to pay for or what gives the dentist the greatest return on time, effort, and materials. The patient, as the consumer, weighs needs and discomfort against the cost of the purchase of dental services. A dentist with a new technique in esthetic dentistry would present it in such a way as to attract patients and build his or her business, thereby keeping it from other dentist competitors. In this model all dentists are in competition, selling the same commodity to the public for the best price, creating a true marketplace. In this commercial model no obligation exists between the dentist, the patient, other dentists, or the community.

Guild Model

The second model, the guild model, presents dentistry as an all-knowing profession. It is called the *guild* model because it resembles the medieval guild of old in which those who were members of the group controlled knowledge, skill, and competency. In this model the patient has dental needs and the dentist, as a member of the profession, provides care to meet the needs of that patient, who is uninformed and passive in the process. This is a paternalistic undertaking in which the obligation to provide care comes from the dentist's membership in his or her chosen profession.

Interactive Model

In the third model, the interactive model, the patient and the dentist are equals and have roles of equal moral status in the process of dental care delivery. According to this model patients determine their own needs and health care choices on the basis of their personal values and priorities but seek the care of the dentist because of his or her knowledge and skill. Thus the status of the dentist and the patient is essentially equal; however, their equality is based on their distinctive roles. Patients needing services and dentists who are able to provide those services are both bound by the common *values* of health and comfort. The obligation for care in this relationship holds both parties as equals because neither can achieve these values without the other. A delicate balance must be maintained in this model between the expertise of the professional and the choice of the patient based on the patient's own values and purposes. Ozar[10] describes this subtle partnership in decision making as the dental professional's first responsibility. The fundamental obligation in the interactive model is for the dentist to treat each patient well and to support the profession. This obligation derives from the larger community sanction that is granted upon graduation and licensure and that is voluntarily accepted upon entrance into the profession.

The three Ozar models provide insight into the moral basis of the relationship of patient and provider in dental care. The interactive model is preferable because it presents the patient and provider as partners who make different contributions to the partnership. This equal moral status creates an obligation for equal respect as partners working together toward attaining and maintaining oral health.

Competency in Dental Hygiene

A basic attribute of professionals is that they have achieved *competency* in the scope of practice that is legally granted to that particular discipline or field. Competencies are essential skills requiring knowledge, skill, and ability that are performed by a health care provider.[11] For a dental hygienist, competencies are skills regularly used in real practice settings to meet the oral health needs of patients. In addition, these competencies have been examined and endorsed by dental hygienists, dentists, and dental educators as valid and appropriate.

The Commission on Dental Accreditation, which is the authorized agency that accredits all dental hygiene education programs in the United States, publishes standards and competencies that all dental hygiene programs must meet or exceed in their educational programs (Box 1-2).

Accreditation in the United States is a system that has been developed to protect the public welfare and provide standards for the evaluation of educational programs and schools. Regional accrediting agencies examine colleges and universities, whereas specialized accrediting agencies focus on a particular profession or occupation. A specialized accrediting agency recognizes a course of instruction composed of a unique set of skills and knowledge, develops the accreditation standards by which such educational programs are evaluated, conducts evaluation of programs, and publishes a list of accredited programs that meet the national accreditation standards. Accreditation standards are developed in consultation with those affected by the standards, who represent the communities of interest. The Commission on Dental Accreditation is the specialized accrediting agency recognized by the United States Department of Education to accredit programs that provide basic preparation for licensure in dentistry, dental hygiene, and all related dental disciplines.[12] The commission consists of 30 members and includes a representative of the ADHA. The commission uses a peer-review process to ensure that the dental hygiene standards are met in each program, and a formal, on-site review is conducted every 7 years.

Patient care competencies, sometimes called *graduation competencies,* are standards that must be met by graduates of any educational program accredited by the Commission on Dental Accreditation. In states in which

BOX 1-2

Patient Care Competencies: Accreditation Standards for Dental Hygiene Education Programs

The Commission on Dental Accreditation is the agency that conducts the accreditation program for all dental education programs. The Commission is the nationally recognized accrediting body for dentally related fields and receives its authority from acceptance by the dental community and by being recognized by the U.S. Department of Education (USDE). The standards for dental hygiene are reviewed and revised periodically through an open and contributory process that includes representatives from the discipline of dental hygiene. The standards listed below may change because of this on-going cycle of review but will include competencies in the following areas.

Graduates from an entry-level dental hygiene education program must be competent in the following:

1. Providing dental hygiene care for the child, adolescent, adult, and geriatric patient including assessing the treatment needs of special needs patients
2. Providing the dental hygiene process of care, which includes:
   - *Assessment:* The collection and analysis of patient needs and oral health problems including medical and dental histories, vital signs, extraoral and intraoral examination, radiographs, indices, and risk analysis.
   - *Planning:* The establishment of realistic goals and treatment strategies to facilitate optimal oral health. This planning would include the dental hygiene diagnosis and treatment plan.
   - *Implementation of the treatment plan:* Implementation would include periodontal debridement and scaling, pain management, fluoride therapy, application of chemotherapeutic agents and sealants, polishing, health education, and nutritional counseling.
   - *Evaluation and measurement of the goals identified in the treatment plan:* This would also include referral for further dental and medical treatment and careful documentation of all procedures
3. Providing dental hygiene care for all types of periodontal disease, including in patients who exhibit moderate to severe periodontal disease
4. Interacting with all types of populations groups and applying interpersonal and communication skills effectively

(Continued)

BOX 1-2

Patient Care Competencies: Accreditation Standards for Dental Hygiene Education Programs—cont'd

5. Assessing, planning, implementing, and evaluating the health promotion activities of community-based oral health programs
6. Providing life support measures in medical emergencies when necessary
7. Applying ethical, legal, and regulatory concepts in the provision of oral health care
8. Identifying self-assessment skills for lifelong learning and improvement of dental hygiene care rendered to patients
9. Evaluating current scientific literature to maintain knowledge of dental hygiene
10. Applying problem-solving strategies in the comprehensive care and management of patients

Based on data from Commission on Dental Accreditation: Accreditation standards for dental hygiene education programs, *Chicago, American Dental Association.*
NOTE: *The newest version of this document is currently under review and expected to be finalized in 2009; however, the basic patient care competencies will remain.*

mastery of additional skills is mandated by the dental practice act, accredited programs also offer training opportunities in those competencies. An example of such a skill or function is the administration of local anesthesia or nitrous oxide analgesia.

Acquisition of dental hygiene skills is a process guided by educational theory and experienced dental hygiene educators. General education, biomedical science, dental science, and dental hygiene science content areas provide the core of knowledge in a dental hygiene program. Educational theory categorizes the process of skill performance into five stages of competency, also termed *the expert learning continuum* (Figure 1-1). The five stages are novice, advanced beginner, competency, proficiency, and expertise.[13,14]

*E*ducation is not the filling of a bucket, but the lighting of a fire.

W.B. YEATS

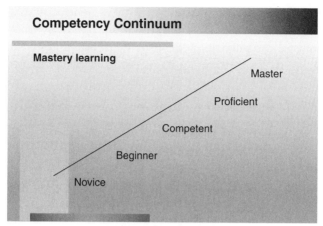

FIGURE 1-1   Competency continuum.

When a student begins preclinical activities and progresses to caring for clinical patients under the supervision of faculty, that stage of learning is called *novice* or *advanced beginner*. At or even before graduation the student will have achieved competency, that is, the ability to perform skills without faculty supervision and with confidence. After graduation, the dental hygienist works toward proficiency and continues working, throughout his or her professional life, toward becoming an expert. Becoming an expert is not an end point; rather it is something a true professional constantly strives for in practice. An analogy is the professional athlete who constantly practices a sport, seeking improvement and even greater ability. Perhaps that is why the term *practice* is used, as in the practice of dental hygiene or the practice of dentistry. Professionals constantly seek to perform at increasingly higher levels, perfecting the art and science of dental hygiene for every patient treated.

▪ Standards for Clinical Practice

The ADHA established **standards** for clinical dental hygiene practice in 1985 to outline the expectations for the practicing dental hygienist.[15] In its role as the organized voice for dental hygiene, the ADHA advocates quality care, health promotion, and enhanced oral health, with the ultimate goal of improving overall health for all individuals and groups. The revised Standards for Clinical Dental Hygiene Practice lay out a framework for clinical practice that focuses on the provision of patient-centered comprehensive care.[16] The six standards of practice are assessment, dental hygiene diagnosis, planning, implementation, evaluation, and documentation (Box 1-3). Establishing, reviewing, revising, and publishing these standards are professional responsibilities that the ADHA assumes for its members to ensure that professional practice is based on the best and most scientifically accurate evidence and practice approaches.

Professional Traits for the Dental Hygienist

The *professional traits* or attributes of a successful dental hygienist are found in the basics of professionalism. These traits are nurtured in the dental hygiene student and then carried into clinical practice or other practice settings.

The attributes that have been identified as those of a health care professional are the same whether that individual is a physician, nurse, dentist, dental hygienist, or other allied health care provider. All these traits are rooted in beneficence: the core of health care that places the needs of the patient or client ahead of those of the provider. Society expects and demands this behavior from individuals who choose to pursue a career in the health fields. From the perspective of the general population, the term *professional* has evolved to mean an individual who demonstrates certain attributes, *traits,* and behaviors that embrace the best qualities of care and service.

The ethicist Laurence McCullough has stated that two virtues are required in a professional person. The first is self-effacement, which means putting aside all notions of self as better educated, socially superior, or more economically well off and focusing on the needs of the patient. The second is self-sacrifice, or putting aside or giving up one's own interests and concerns.

The professional traits that a dental hygienist must demonstrate and a dental hygiene student should strive to develop are listed in Box 1-4 and discussed in the following section. Dental hygienists who demonstrate these traits will experience a positive level of satisfaction in the practice of dental hygiene and will be able to recognize their contributions to the overall benefit of society.

Honesty and Integrity

A relationship of trust is essential to providing care when personal health information is shared. The patient should be confident that information given in written and verbal form is held in confidence and handled appropriately.

BOX 1-3

Highlights of the Standards for Clinical Dental Hygiene Practice*

Standard 1: Assessment
Assessment is the systematic collection, analysis, and documentation of oral and general health status and patient needs. It is comprised of patient history collection, performing a clinical evaluation, and measuring risk assessment.

Standard 2: Dental Hygiene Diagnosis
The dental hygiene diagnosis is a component of the overall dental diagnosis. It is the identification of an existing or potential oral health problem that the hygienist is educationally qualified and licensed to treat. This aspect of practice involves analyzing and interpreting all data to determine the patient need and how the diagnosis is incorporated into the overall dental treatment plan.

Standard 3: Planning
The plan of care is based on the assessment and dental hygiene diagnosis and establishes the goals and outcomes based on patient needs, expectations, and evidence.

Standard 4: Implementation
The delivery of dental hygiene services to the patient is the implementation aspect of practice. Modification of care often occurs to minimize risk, thus optimizing the outcome of the care plan.

Standard 5: Evaluation
Evaluation is the process of reviewing and documenting the outcomes of dental hygiene care. Measurable criteria are used to judge the results of treatment approaches.

Standard 6: Documentation
The accurate recording of collected data, treatment planned and provided during patient care, is entered to create a permanent document. This information is recorded appropriately and should meet all state regulations and ethical guidelines.

Data from American Dental Hygienists' Association: Standards for clinical dental hygiene practice, *Chicago, 2008, Author.*
Full text available at: www.adha.org/downloads/adha_standardso8.pdf. Accessed September 4, 2008.

BOX 1-4

Professional Traits of the Dental Hygienist

- Honesty and integrity
- Caring and compassion
- Reliability and responsibility
- Maturity and self-analysis
- Loyalty
- Interpersonal communication
- Respect for others
- Respect for self

Patients and colleagues must be able to depend on the words and actions of individuals who treat and work with them. Professional integrity is a commitment to upholding the Code of Ethics and the standards of care.

I've learned that making a "living" is not the same as making a "life."

MAYA ANGELOU

Caring and Compassion

The ability to care for and be compassionate to each and every patient is a critical trait expected of all individuals who seek a career in a health care profession. Caring means demonstrating the empathy necessary to comfort and guide the patient in the health promotion process. Persons who are compassionate are merciful to all patients, including those who are unlike themselves or who are possibly difficult to understand and treat.

Reliability and Responsibility

The dental hygienist must accept responsibility for performing all services to the best standard of care. Sound judgment must be applied in every patient encounter, keeping in mind the technical, scientific, and ethical dimensions of the case. Maintaining current knowledge of dental hygiene theory and technique is part of that responsibility. Most states have a legal requirement for continuing education for those who hold a dental hygiene or dental license. The goal of mandated continuing education is to ensure optimal health services to the public by fostering continued competence. A reliable individual meets the obligations of time and duty, keeping appointments and meeting established schedules.

> *I believe that every right implies a responsibility; every opportunity, an obligation; every possession, a duty.*
>
> JOHN D. ROCKEFELLER

Maturity and Self-Analysis

A mature individual works efficiently and effectively toward the goals of attaining and maintaining oral health for each patient. The dental hygienist often seeks employment in solo or group dental practices in which a small number of individuals must work as a team, relying on each person to perform his or her assigned role and to always keep the needs of the patient primary to all activities. Self-analysis is the trait in which the dental hygienist assesses his or her skills and takes responsibility for changing and improving those skills when necessary.

> *The only person who is educated is the one who has learned how to learn and change.*
>
> CARL ROGERS

Loyalty

Protecting and promoting the interests of a person, group, or organization is the definition of loyalty. Any relationship between a health care provider and a patient is a special affiliation; all professional decisions must be unencumbered by conflicting personal interests. Promises should be carefully made and kept.

Interpersonal Communication

The foundation of trust lies in communication and the ability of the patient to speak and be heard. Listening to the overt and subtle cues provided by patients allows the dental hygienist to develop a relationship that fosters an open exchange of information. Patients expect that personal, intimate facts and impressions about them will be kept in confidence by the dental hygienist.

Tolerance for Others

To treat all patients without discrimination is a basic ethical and legal requirement. This behavior goes beyond the legal warning to not discriminate based on race, creed, color, age, sex, ethnicity, or disabilities to include occupation, financial status, personality, and oral conditions. It means caring for all individuals who seek treatment whether or not they are likeable. Patients occasionally will prove difficult and hostile during the course of treatment, but the dental hygienist must still treat them to the best of his or her ability.

Respect for Self

Dental hygienists should maintain their own physical and mental health so that the patient's needs can remain the primary focus. Working while under the influence of alcohol, drugs, lack of sleep, or emotional distress does not allow the health care provider to focus on the needs of the patient. Each patient deserves the complete attention of the dental hygienist while being treated.

> **W**hat you are thunders so loudly that I cannot hear what you say to the contrary.
>
> RALPH WALDO EMERSON

Legal Requirements for the Dental Hygienist

Dental hygienists are subject to the rules and regulations of the jurisdiction in which they practice dental hygiene. When a license is granted to an individual, that person becomes responsible for knowing and upholding all the statutes and laws set down in the legal document, usually called the *state dental practice act* or the *code of dental practice.* Ignorance of a portion of the law or code is no excuse for noncompliance by a dental hygienist or any other health care provider. The responsibility and power for legislative protection of the public rest with each individual state or territory. **Licensure** is designed to enforce practice codes, establish standards, and sanction incompetent practitioners, all for the purpose of protecting the health and safety of the public.

The scope of practice of a dental hygienist was first established by law in Connecticut in 1915 at the urging of Dr. A.C. Fones, the father of dental hygiene. The Connecticut dental law delineated the practice parameters of the dental hygienist and subsequently served as a model for the states that later adopted similar legislation. All state boards, as well as those in the Virgin Islands and Puerto Rico, grant a license to practice to the dental hygienist. An unlicensed person may not provide dental hygiene care.

Legal statutes periodically change in response to many factors, both to protect the public and advance the interests of the health professions. The process for any legal change is arduous, complicated, and costly in time and effort. Most legislative changes related to dental health care are driven by individuals in the dental and dental hygiene professions. For the most part the public remains unaware of the intricacies of the process or its effect on their dental health care delivery. Some of the factors that influence legislative changes in a state include the following:

- Need and demand for dental care
- Distribution of dental health care providers
- Federal health legislation
- Goals of organized dental and dental hygiene associations advocacy groups

Increases in the scope of practice for the dental hygienist have occurred over the years but usually have been accompanied by a great deal of controversy and consternation. The services performed by the dental hygienist usually are classified as either traditional duties, such as scaling, root planing, and education of the patient, or expanded functions, such as the administration of local anesthesia and placement of restorative materials. Some states have implemented an additional practice level for dental hygienists, termed an *expanded-* or *extended-duty dental hygienist.* Individuals pursuing this level of practice must complete additional training in periodontal or restorative functions and be sanctioned to perform these skills by the particular state in which they practice. The specific duties of the dental hygienist in a given state are detailed in the dental statutes or dental practice act. Only duties or functions allowed in a particular state may be performed by the licensed dental hygienist, even if that individual is trained and licensed in another state where the practice act is more expansive. The exact duties and services that may be performed by the dental hygienist in a particular state are based on customary parameters of practice and the state dental practice act.

The legal mandates in each state use terms that differentiate the level of supervision set out by that particular body. Some states are more liberal in their dental practice acts than others. Several states have adopted mechanisms to allow a dental hygienist to practice without the supervision of a dentist after gaining a special license or credential. These allowances are granted after additional training or testing, often with the goal of improving public access to appropriate care.

■ Summary

The profession of dental hygiene was established with the goal of providing oral health education and services to the public so that dental disease could be prevented. As a health care professional, the dental hygienist is given the trust of society; with that special trust come rights and responsibilities. Attaining and maintaining competency in dental hygiene are among the obligations that the dental hygienist accepts in completing a formal education program and passing the state licensure examination. The traits that characterize a successful dental hygienist are the same traits found in any successful health care professional: placing the needs of the patient first and aiming to provide the best care to every patient as well as society at large.

REFERENCES

1 Steele PF: *Dimensions of dental hygiene,* ed 3, Philadelphia, 1983, Lea & Febiger, p 477.
2 Deleted.
3 Motley WE: *Ethics, jurisprudence and history for the dental hygienist,* ed 3, Philadelphia, 1983, Lea & Febiger.
4 Beemsterboer PL: Developing an ethic of access to care in dentistry, *J Dent Educ* 70(11):1212, 2006.
5 Medical professionalism in the new millennium: a physician charter, *Ann Intern Med* 136(3):36, 2002.
6 Ring ME: *Dentistry: an illustrated history,* New York, 1992, H. Abrams.
7 Brint S: *In an age of experts: the changing role of professionals in politics and public life,* Princeton, NJ, 1994, Princeton University Press.

8 Sullivan WM: *Work and integrity,* ed 2, San Francisco, 2005, Jossey-Bass.

9 Stern DT: *Measuring medical professionalism,* New York, 2006, Oxford University Press.

10 Ozar DT: Three models of professionalism and professional obligation in dentistry, *J Am Dent Assoc* 110:173, 1985.

11 Beemsterboer PL: Competency in allied dental education, *J Dent Educ* 11:19, 1994.

12 Commission on Dental Accreditation: *Accreditation standards for dental hygiene education programs,* Chicago, 1998, American Dental Association, Available at www.ada.org/prof/ed/accred/standards/dh_08.pdf. Accessed September 4, 2008.

13 Chambers DW: Toward a competency-based curriculum, *J Dent Educ* 57:790, 1993.

14 Chi MT, Glaser R, Farr M: *The nature of expertise,* Hillsdale, NJ, 1988, Lawrence Erlbaum.

15 American Dental Hygienists' Association: *Standards of applied dental hygiene practice,* Chicago, 1985, Author.

16 American Dental Hygienists' Association: *Standards for clinical dental hygiene practice,* Chicago, 2008, Author. Available at www.adha.org/downloads/adha_standards08.pdf. Accessed September 4, 2008.

CHAPTER 2

Ethical Theory and Philosophy

PHYLLIS L. BEEMSTERBOER AND DAVID OZAR

LEARNING OUTCOMES

- Explain the main components of moral growth.
- Describe the theories of moral development and the role of cognitive growth.
- Discuss character and the contribution of character development to ethical conduct for the health care provider.
- Compare the three theories of ethical thinking and give examples of each from oral health care.

KEY TERMS

amoral

autonomous

character

consequentialism

ethical theory

ethics

morality

moral reasoning

nonconsequentialism

utilitarianism

virtue ethics

As a health care provider, the dental hygienist will be faced with numerous professional and personal problems. Differences exist between addressing everyday problems and addressing ethical dilemmas. To reach this understanding, an introduction to the foundation of ethical theory is important to guide ethical decision making as well as assist in understanding the process by which such decisions are made. Ethical decision making is a behavior and, as a behavior, is something that can be taught and learned. Thus this chapter begins with an overview of moral development and then examines three broad approaches from moral philosophy that should enhance the understanding of how **ethical theory** lays the foundation for ethical decision making. Chapter 3 builds on ethical theory by introducing conceptual tools that can be applied in real-life situations.

The key to your universe is that you can choose.

CARL FREDERICK

Moral Development

How do individuals become moral? Are we born moral, or do we learn to be moral? If **morality** is something that must be learned, how is it learned? Do all persons learn morality at the same rate and to the same degree? If human beings are born capable of becoming moral and therefore must learn to be moral, how do individuals learn to differentiate right from wrong and how do they incorporate this skill in life?

Several authors have focused on moral development as a process. Just as each individual develops physically and intellectually, moral development also has been shown to typically occur in progressive steps or stages. Some researchers have related age, maturation of components of personality, and increased experience with moral development, whereas others have stressed that moral development has a cognitive component as well. That is why differentiating right from wrong, which is a cognitive matter, is different from incorporating right and wrong into life—that is, moral development overall. The examples of saints and heroes, as well as moral growth by ordinary people every day, can give clues about the causes or mechanisms of moral development. Psychological research on moral development is a fairly new field and, from a scientific point of view, much of what is involved remains unclear.

What has become clear is that a strong relationship exists between education and development of moral judgment, the cognitive aspect of moral development. One of the strongest and most consistent correlates with development of moral judgment, even stronger than chronologic age, is years of formal education.[1,2] It seems that moral development continues as long as person is in a formal education environment and typically plateaus upon leaving school. This is an important lesson. If you want to keep growing as a moral human being, keep learning; keep observing and reflecting on what is going on around you and keep asking questions, read and discuss with others to keep these activities vital, and above all do so in aspects of your life in which moral matters are at stake. Professional life obviously is one of those aspects.

Various educational programs and interventions have been used to facilitate development of moral judgment by providing enriched and stimulating educational experiences. A review of moral education programs revealed that almost half were effective in promoting moral development, especially if the program lasted longer than a few weeks and if the program involved the participants in discussions of controversial moral dilemmas.[3] Adults also seemed to gain more from such programs than did younger children.

These findings have implications for persons preparing for a career in dental hygiene because they emphasize several things about learning to make moral decisions. First, findings suggest that the capacity for moral judgment is not as rigid as some have argued. That is, a person's cognitive moral development is not frozen at some specified age. Rather, individuals can continue to learn, and research has shown that adults make greater gains than children. Second, individuals in formal education programs will likely benefit from advanced training, especially when expected to test ethical decision-making ability by considering a variety of dental hygiene case scenarios. Third, these findings suggest that participation in continuing education courses after graduation may reinforce an individual's ability to make sound ethics judgments and also have a positive impact on the person's commitment to practicing in an ethical manner.

▪ Theories of Cognitive Moral Development

Male Justice Orientation

Moral development has been studied a great deal by psychologists, who have provided some knowledge of the process and how it influences our actions in adulthood. The most famous developmental psychologists, Piaget[4] and Kohlberg,[5] categorized stages in the moral development of male children. Piaget and Kohlberg both stated that moral development is sequential and depends on an individual's level of cognitive development. Piaget's[4] model consisted of four stages (Table 2-1), whereas Kohlberg[5] defined moral development according to both levels and stages (Table 2-2).

Each stage in the process of cognitive moral development involves judgment skills that are more complex, comprehensive, and differentiated from the preceding stage. The process also is sequential, with an individual moving from simple to more complex stages. Kohlberg's stages follow the Piagetian view that justice is the core of morality; but because this was first demonstrated empirically only in male subjects, it is important not to generalize more broadly at this point. Kohlberg's theory focuses primarily on cognitive

TABLE 2-1
Piaget's Four-Stage Model of Moral Development

STAGE	CHARACTERISTICS OF MORAL DEVELOPMENT
1	*Amoral* stage (ages 0 to 2 years)
2	Egocentric stage (ages 2 to 7 years); bends rules and reacts to environment instinctively
3	Heteronomous stage (ages 7 to 12 years); accepts the moral authority of others
4	*Autonomous* stage (ages 12 and older); a morality of self based on cooperation; rules tested and become internalized

TABLE 2-2
Kohlberg's Three-Level Model of Moral Development

LEVEL	LEVEL OF REASONING	STAGE
1	Preconventional reasoning (stages 1 and 2), in which externally established rules determine right and wrong action	Stage 1: punishment and obedience orientation Stage 2: instrumental relativist orientation
2	Conventional reasoning (stages 3 and 4), in which expectations of family and groups are maintained and where loyalty and conformity are considered important	Stage 3: interpersonal concordance orientation Stage 4: law and order orientation
3	Postconventional or principled (stages 5 and 6), in which the person autonomously examines and defines moral values with decisions of conscience dictating the right action	Stage 5: social contract legalistic orientation Stage 6: universal ethical principle orientation

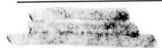

processes, which is consistent with his belief that thought guides behavior. He asserts the moral superiority of his stage 6, where what he considers to be genuine moral judgments are made. Genuine moral judgments are defined as judgments about the good and right of actions based on objective, impersonal, or ideal grounds.[6] Thus cognitive moral development is a progression toward increasingly valid or universal moral thought. The health care provider ideally should be able to make genuine moral judgments even if there is more to cognitive moral development than Kohlberg has discussed.

Female Ethic of Care

Among the criticisms of Kohlberg's work is the challenge that his model reflects a male-oriented perspective of morality. Gilligan,[7] in her classic book, states that women tend to see morality in the context of a relationship she calls the *ethic of care*. She explains that feminine moral reasoning is different from masculine moral reasoning. To survive evolutionarily and practically, female individuals have had to develop a sense of responsibility based on the universal principle of caring, which Gilligan sees as quite different from universal justice. Like Kohlberg's model, Gilligan's model also has three levels (Table 2-3).

Gilligan believes that complete moral development occurs in the context of two moral orientations—a male justice orientation and a female ethic of care—and therefore that Kohlberg's measurement of moral development *only* in a justice-oriented scoring system is biased toward the male. Gilligan's work, which focuses on gender differences within the study of moral judgment development, has received much interest and support.[8] As an oversimplified example of her model, the male health care provider, when discovering a case of suspected child abuse, would acknowledge his duty to report, report the suspicious case, and move on. For the female health care provider, however, the duty to report is derived from the relationships

TABLE 2-3

Gilligan's Model of Moral Development

LEVEL	CARE ORIENTATION
1	Orientation to individual survival and being moral is surviving by being submissive to society
2	Goodness as self-sacrifice, in which being moral is first not hurting others with no thought of hurt to self
3	Morality of nonviolence; avoiding hurt becomes the moral guide governing all moral reasoning

surrounding the child and the need to protect the interests of the child. Her actions might well be identical with those of the male, but the basis of their being ethically required would be different. One reason for this difference in Gilligan's theory of moral development is that it is based on the way girls are raised. The care orientation is a parallel path of moral development and perhaps one that will provide further insight into justice orientation. But in any case, in this text both perspectives are accepted a crucial to the understanding of moral development.

Cognitive Development Theory

The basic tenet of cognitive development theory is that people operate on their experiences to make sense of them, and those experiences, as we make sense of them, in turn change the basic conceptual structures by which people construct meanings. Researchers studying the relation between moral judgment and behavior assume that many factors determine behavior. For example, studies link moral perception with actual, real-life behavior as well as moral judgment. In addition, the literature suggests that students pursuing professional education are "in an important formative period of ethical development and that formal schooling is a powerful catalyst to ethical development."[9] Rest[10] and his co-workers have explained this by saying that people who develop in moral judgment are those who love to learn; seek challenges; and are reflective, set goals, take risks, and profit from stimulating and challenging environments. These are characteristics frequently found in professional students who are working hard to become excellent professionals.

Nurture your mind with great thoughts, for you will never go any higher than you think.

BENJAMIN DISRAELI

■ Character

The issue of *character* in an individual and the process of character education are topics that have gained significant attention in recent years, primarily because of a perceived lack of character development in today's society. Character usually is defined as qualities or dispositions that are consistently practiced. The term comes from a Greek term meaning a constellation of strengths and weaknesses that form the person.

Some colleges and several philanthropic foundations have established character development or a character focus as their mission. One such example is the Josephson Institute of Ethics, based in Marina Del Rey, Calif. This nonprofit group supports character-based decision making using consequentialist and virtue philosophy. Their basic program is called the "Character Counts Coalition," and it includes six core ethical values: (1) trustworthiness, (2) respect, (3) responsibility, (4) fairness, (5) caring, and (6) citizenship. The mission of the Josephson Institute is to improve the ethical quality of society by teaching principled reasoning and ethical decision making. Programs are targeted at children in schools; legislators; lawyers; journalists; and leaders in the corporate, public, and nonprofit sectors. Another example is the Templeton Foundation, in Radnor, Penn., which sponsors character education programs. All these efforts are grounded in the belief that positive traits of character can be forged through educational experiences, whether in elementary or high school or professional school. They also presume that character can be shaped and influenced by good example at every level of learning.

The reason for mentioning character here is twofold. First, as stressed above, the cognitive aspects of moral development are only part of the story. Incorporating the skill of differentiating right from wrong into life is a matter of building habits—habits of carefully judging as well as carefully perceiving and consistently acting in accordance with one's moral judgments. One of the best ways to appreciate the value of a habit is to see how it operates in someone we admire, which is why good examples are so important to moral development. But on the cognitive side, which is the focus of this chapter, much can be learned; a focus on the different ways in which moral thinking can be done, so one can come to a well-reasoned moral judgment, is an important first step. In the academic world, examining the different ways in which moral thinking can be done is called a *study of moral or ethical theory.* To keep matters simple, an "ethical" or "moral" question (compared with a question that has nothing to do with ethics or morality) is a question in which a person's well-being or rights or duties are at issue or at stake. In addition, because the meanings of "ethical" and "moral" are not carefully distinguished in a manner that is widely and consistently used, these terms often are treated as synonyms and used interchangeably.

*P*ride is concerned with who is right. Humility is concerned with what is right.

EZRA TAFT BENSON

Be more concerned with your character than your reputation, because your character is what you really are, while your reputation is merely what others think you are.

JOHN WOODEN

Overview of Ethical Theories

The role of ethical theories is to lay a foundation for ethical decision making. A system of *moral reasoning* or moral thinking is important because it provides a frame of reference that will help the individual make morally appropriate responses to moral dilemmas.

Although multiple theories have been proposed to explain how people direct their actions when faced with a moral dilemma, three broad-based classical views or philosophies comprising *ethics* are reviewed. The three views or philosophies that comprise ethical theory are consequentialism, deontology or nonconsequentialism, and virtue ethics.[11] A brief overview of these approaches is presented to acquaint the reader with some of the assumptions, beliefs, and traditions underlying thought and action.

Consequentialism or Utilitarian Ethics

CONSEQUENTIALIST ETHICS

An action or rule is right insofar as it produces or leads to the maximization of good consequences.

Consequentialism is predicated on the idea that the rightness or wrongness of any action is determined and justified by the consequences of the act judged in comparison with other possible acts that might be performed in the situation. Consequentialist thinking is always comparative because it aims at maximizing good consequences (and minimizing harmful ones). Thus consequentialists consider the consequences of each important alternative course of action available to them in the situation before deciding on a right action. Such individuals consider all relevant consequences (potential outcomes) of an action before making a choice about which action to take, believing that, if a person can identify and evaluate (in terms of benefit and harm) all the consequences, making a choice about which action or actions are right actions is possible; namely, the action(s) that, compared with the alternatives, yield the best outcomes.

For example, a dental hygienist may observe that her employer routinely leaves overhangs on restored teeth. Because overhangs may negatively affect the patient's periodontal health, the hygienist must determine what, if any, action to take. She begins by identifying her alternatives and examining the benefit or harm that will most likely result from each one. First, the hygienist could take no action. One consequence of inaction might result in some patients developing severe periodontal disease and/or losing teeth. Second, the hygienist could remove the overhangs. One consequence of this action would be enhanced oral health for the patient. However, in some states removal of overhangs may be illegal for a hygienist, and doing so could put her professional reputation in jeopardy or anger the dentist. Third, the hygienist could discuss with the employer the fact that overhangs are frequently present. The consequences could be that the dentist would restore teeth more carefully. However, another consequence might be that the dentist simply tells the hygienist to mind her own business and do her job. If the hygienist persists, the employer may decide to terminate employment. All these are consequences to consider because they are important alternatives for the dental hygienist in this situation. However, notice that the consequential reasoning approach would require the hygienist to do what is good even when it might not be in the hygienist's own best interest. Being ethical is not always easy. On the other hand, another action not considered here might maximize everyone's best interests. This is why consequentialist thinking must involve a careful look at all the alternative actions available and evaluate their consequences for good and for harm very carefully before determining which maximizes the good (and minimizes the harm).

John Stuart Mill was one of the most famous proponents of **utilitarianism,** a theory also based on the consequentialist approach to decision making. He stressed that, in consequentialist reasoning, every person affected by an action should be considered.[11] Mill often is described as saying that an action should be judged to be moral on its capacity to provide the greatest good for the largest number of people. However, his teacher Bentham said that, not Mill, and Mill eventually repudiated the phrase because it misled people into thinking that, for a utilitarian, whatever benefitted the *majority* was the right thing to do. Both men did teach that the moral action is the one (of the alternative actions available) that maximizes good and minimizes harm when the consequences for every affected person are considered. Consequences may be considered on an individual basis, but utilitarianism stresses that they must be considered for everyone affected. Obviously one place where utilitarian reasoning might be appropriate is when ethical matters must be decided (e.g., by a legislator or officer of government) that affect large social systems, a community, or even a nation. A public health dentist or a hygienist with a master's degree in public health would be more likely to use this approach in public health thinking than would others. Thus one of the best examples of utilitarianism in dentistry is the application of fluoride to community water systems. The consequence was a benefit through caries reduction, provided at a relatively low cost and available to all members of a community regardless of social status or income, and with almost no possibility of causing harm. The alternative was one in which many people had many more carious lesions and other dental problems because their oral hygiene was not dependable enough to prevent these harms.

Deontology or Nonconsequentialism

NONCONSEQUENTIALIST ETHICS

The central claim of deontological or nonconsequentialist ethics is that an action is right when it conforms to a principle or rule of conduct that meets a requirement of some overriding duty.

The expression *deontological ethics* is derived from the Greek word *deon*, meaning duty. Deontologists state that some actions are required by the rightness or wrongness of the action, regardless of the consequences of the action. Whereas consequentialists focus on the consequences of an act, deontologists argue that some acts are right or wrong independent of their consequences (thus the term **nonconsequentialism**). Some acts are right because they have a direct relation to some overriding duty, or they are wrong because they directly violate some overriding duty, but not because of consequences. For example, a deontologist might believe that a health care provider, as a moral person, has a duty to tell the truth in all circumstances and therefore has a specific duty to tell the truth to patients. With this view, a professional's duty to tell the truth to a patient is not founded on the consequences of telling the patient the truth, but on the belief either that an absolute duty exists never to lie or that the patient is entitled by reason of a fundamental right to receive the truth. According to deontology, then, moral standards exist independently of the particular circumstances of an action and do not depend on consequences. Duty and the relation of a person's actions to duty are the only relevant considerations.

Immanuel Kant[12] is credited for establishing one of the most detailed nonconsequentialist or deontological theories of ethical thinking. Kant held that the test of any rule of conduct is whether it can be a duty for all human beings to act on—what he called a *universal law.* That test is, for Kant, what tells us whether an action is directly related to an overriding duty. Kant also stressed that all human beings (as adults) are free, are worthy of respect, and are their own choosers of their purposes and actions. Many deontological theories of human rights have been built by later thinkers on this basis.[12] This school of thought has had a significant effect on biomedical ethics. It places primacy on the right of the individual to act autonomously, that is, to make his or her own decisions on the basis of his or her own values, goals, principles, and ideals. Autonomy as an important principle of health care ethics is further explored in Chapter 3.

Kant's test was called *the categorical imperative,* which means a rule or standard of conduct that is absolutely binding for all human beings under all circumstances in which the rule or standard applies. Kant held that some of the moral rules we are familiar with (e.g., do not lie) have this character of overriding duty. Most of the rules with this character are negative, in that they tell a person what *not* to do. For example, one must not lie, cheat, or steal. Borrowing an old Latin word, *perfectum,* which meant "binding unconditionally," Kant categorized the negative rules having this character as "perfect duties." Perfect duties are always binding. Kant also talked about "imperfect duties," which refer to moral obligations to act in certain ways during our lives but leave it to each person to judge when and in what situation to fulfill the obligation (*imperfect* here meaning "conditionally binding," that is, depending on the actor's judgment to determine when to fulfill the obligation). Thus a perfect duty requires one not to kill an innocent human being. The prohibition against murder is binding because it is right and directly connected to an overriding duty, not because of the consequences. According to this perfect duty, one person cannot morally kill another person even if such an act was the only possible way to save the lives of others. Not stealing also is a perfect duty. An imperfect duty is an obligation to help another person in need or to be compassionate. We all have an overriding duty to attend to people's needs, but we are not obligated to try to meet them in every situation in which someone is in need. It is a matter of moral judgment that a person must carefully make to determine for whom and in which situations to fulfill this duty.[12]

Sometimes Kant's categoric imperative is compared with the golden rule, which cautions individuals to "do unto others as you would have others do unto you." As Kant stated it, "Act that you can will the maxim of your action to be a universal law binding upon the will of every other rationale person."[12]

An example of the deontological approach as it applies to dental hygiene is that a hygienist has a duty to maintain patient confidentiality except in the provision of oral health care for her patient. Other than sharing information appropriately with other health care providers, information acquired while providing patient care must remain private unless the patient's express permission has been granted. If an adult patient's relative or a representative of a finance company asks questions regarding the patient, confidentiality must be maintained. It is right because respect for others' autonomy is an overriding duty, and a patient's revelation of personal information to the hygienist for purposes of oral health care does not include permission to use it for any other purpose. If this philosophy were strictly held in health care, public health reporting of communicable disease would seem to not be permitted. However, Kant expanded his moral theory to cover societal rules in ways that could make such reporting morally acceptable if one could reasonably argue that any rational person would want such information communicated to avoid harm to others. Just as consequentialist thinking can get quite complex when many alternative actions must be compared, when consequences are hard to predict, and when different kinds of benefits and harms affect different persons as a consequence of an action, so deontological thinking—though it may appear simple at the start—can be complex when trying to determine what social standards could reasonably be willed by rational people to be universal standards to live by. No moral philosopher has ever claimed that moral thinking is like solving a simple equation in mathematics. One reason theories have been offered is to help us understand how complex making good moral decisions can be, and then to try to help us think about them more clearly.

Let us have faith that right makes might, and in that faith let us in the end dare to do our duty as we understand it.

ABRAHAM LINCOLN

Virtue Ethics

VIRTUE ETHICS

Character or virtue and the goodness of the person in living a good life, acquired by a person through learning and reflection and repetition (based on Greek tradition of Plato and Aristotle).

Character, or virtue, refers to stable patterns of perceiving, thinking, and acting rightly. A person cannot stop and carefully weigh possible actions in terms of ethical standards hundreds of times a day even though hundreds of opportunities for action each day are ethically significant. Therefore most of our actions are the product of our character, or the stable patterns perceiving, thinking, and acting that are part of us. If those patterns are perceiving, thinking, and acting rightly we call them *virtues* and we say the person has a "good character" or is a "good person." And when we speak of professionalism in any profession, we are talking about stable patterns of perceiving, thinking, and acting in accord with the profession's ethical standards. Character and virtue therefore are central themes in any discussion of ethics for professionals.

Virtue ethics was first articulated as a moral theory in the Greek tradition of Plato and Aristotle, who emphasized that the cultivation of virtuous traits of character is the primary function of morality. Aristotle wrote that virtue is a stable state of character and is the result of practice— that virtue is something acquired by a person through learning, reflection, and repetition. When trying to describe the virtues of good persons, he looked for a balance between intellect and commitment in action (just as moral development is understood today to involve both cognitive and noncognitive components). He also stressed that the person who is virtuous has developed the ability to perceive, judge, and act rightly as a dependable habit; the ideal is stability in these patterns so that the virtuous person would act in a virtuous manner in all situations. Aristotle also recognized that we are all fallible in achieving this ideal and stressed the value for each of us to identify role models whom we can learn from to become more virtuous and do the right thing in each situation more easily and regularly.

Each of the virtues is a habitual disposition to perceive, judge, and act rightly. Virtue ethics focuses not so much on the rightness or wrongness of a given act or whether it conforms to duty, but rather on the goodness of the person who habitually chooses to act in that way or see such acts as proper responses to duty.[13] Rather than focusing first on consequences or nonconsequentialist factors such as duty or rights, philosophers of the virtue ethics tradition urge us to reflect on what kind of person we *ought* to be (and *ought not* be) and not the ethical characteristics of the acts we ought to do. A dental hygienist could treat a hostile and unhappy patient with extra kindness and caring to maximize good and reduce harm or because she considers it her duty. But in the rush of daily professional life, a dental hygienist will more likely do this to be a good professional and a good caring person. When this is her ethical perspective, she clearly is striving to be virtuous but is doing her ethical thinking according to the virtue ethics approach.

Thus virtue ethicists believe that individuals make most of their choices on the basis of virtue and character. The focus is on the character of the person. If a person has good character, that person will make choices that produce good. In an ideal world, of course, all people would be of good character and would make good choices easily and habitually in every situation. But we know that few, if any, of us have completely arrived at that point. Even if, speaking ideally, all people of good character have good ethical decision-making abilities, in the real world we have to work to develop these abilities first and then make them into habitual patterns of perceiving, judging, and acting in our lives.

> Many people say that it is the intellect which makes a great scientist. They are wrong: it is character.
>
> ALBERT EINSTEIN

▉ Summary

Rarely does a person embrace one ethical philosophy exclusively. More than likely an individual is influenced by more than one ethical system as well as by a number of other factors, including religion, culture, and environment. However, knowledge of these philosophical frameworks for ethical thinking helps health care providers understand their professional commitments more clearly and understand their patients and co-workers better as well as their own personal philosophy while dealing with problems and dilemmas in the delivery of health care. The profession of dental hygiene needs people of good character who can, as a result of education, experience, and careful reflection, acquire more skill in making ethical decisions and acting according to them.

REFERENCES

1 Rest JR, Thoma S: The relation of moral judgment development to formal education, *Dev Psychol* 21:709, 1985.

2 Newell KJ, Young LJ, Yamoor CM: Moral reasoning in dental hygiene students, *J Dent Educ* 49:79, 1985.

3 Schlaefli A, Rest J, Thoma S: Does moral education improve moral judgment? A meta-analysis of intervention studies using the defining issues test, *Rev Educ Res* 55:319, 1985.

4 Piaget J [Gabian M, trans]: *The moral judgment of a child*, New York, 1964, The Free Press.

5 Kohlberg L: The cognitive-developmental approach to moral education, In Scharf P, editor: *Readings in moral education*, Minneapolis, 1978, Winston Press.

6 Kohlberg L: Stage and sequence: the cognitive development approach to socialization, In Goslin D, editor: *Handbook of socialization theory and research*, Chicago, 1969, Rand McNally, pp 347-480.

7 Gilligan C: *In a different voice*, Cambridge, Mass, 1982, Harvard University Press.

8 Nokes KM: Rethinking moral reasoning theory, *J Nur Scholar* 21:172, 1989.

9 Rest JR: Can ethics be taught in professional schools? The psychological research. In *Easier said than done*, [newsletter], Marina del Rey, Calif, 1988, Josephson Institute, pp 22-26.

10 Rest JR: *Moral development: advances in research and theory*, New York, 1986, Praeger, p 57.

11 Beauchamp TL, Childress JF: *Principles of biomedical ethics*, ed 4, New York, 1994, Oxford University Press.

12 Kant I [Beck LW, trans]: *Critique of practical reason*, Indianpolis, 1956, Bobbs-Merrill.

13 Ozar DT, Sokol DJ: *Dental ethics at chairside: professional principles and practical Applications*, ed 2, Washington, DC, 2002, Georgetown University Press.

CHAPTER 3

Ethical Principles and Values

PHYLLIS L. BEEMSTERBOER

LEARNING OUTCOMES

- Identify and describe the normative ethical principles.
- Describe the difference between a choice and an ethical dilemma.
- Explain the role of principles in the decision-making process of the dental hygienist.
- Compare the values and ethical concepts that support the principles of ethics.

KEY TERMS

autonomy

beneficence

confidentiality

distributive justice

implied

informed consent

justice

nonmaleficence

paternalism

prima facie duty

primum non nocere

veracity

Ethical principles guide the conduct of health care providers by helping to identify, clarify, and justify moral choices. Principles help address the moral question: What ought I do in the situation I now face? More specifically, what is good, right, or proper for a person to do in this situation? Normative principles provide a cognitive framework for analyzing moral questions and problems. These principles are linked to commonly expected behaviors because they are based on shared standards of thinking and behaving. In health care, the normative principles are nonmaleficence, beneficence, autonomy, and justice. These principles are associated with expectations for behavior, and they provide guidelines in dealing with right and wrong actions. These principles provide direction about what should and should not be done in specific situations.

The very spring and root of honesty and virtue lie in good education.

PLUTARCH

Ethical Dilemmas

A difference exists between addressing everyday problems and addressing ethical dilemmas. What is an ethical dilemma? An ethical dilemma occurs when one or more ethical principles are in conflict. An example of a true ethical dilemma is one in which the principle of nonmaleficence is in conflict with the principle of autonomy in a specific situation. Such a dilemma might occur, for example, when a patient who has undergone heart valve replacement and who requires premedication tells the dental hygienist he does not want to take any antibiotics and urges the dental hygienist to go ahead with scaling and root planing. The patient is expressing his autonomy by stating he does not wish to be premedicated. The dental hygienist, however, has taken an oath to do no harm (nonmaleficence). This is a genuine ethical dilemma because two ethical principles (patient autonomy and nonmaleficence) are in conflict. Resolving an ethical dilemma is certainly a very different enterprise from solving daily problems, such as which automobile to purchase or which instrument to choose for scaling. It also is different from a situation in which a dentist is knowingly and intentionally charging an insurance company for procedures not performed. That clearly involves unethical and unlawful behavior, but it is not a true ethical dilemma because principles are not in conflict. The dentist is wrong and committing fraud. A discussion of which ethical principle takes precedence over another is not necessary. The dentist's behavior is wrong, unjust, and unlawful.

In a perfect world, the needs and wants of the patient would always come first, and no conflicts, disputes, or dilemmas would exist for the dental hygienist or any health care provider to resolve. However, that is not the case in the real world, where what is in the patient's best interest may be open to question depending on whose perspective—that of the clinician, the patient, the patient's family, or other health care professional—is being considered. Principles, values, and rules in health care will help guide decision making in the process of providing the best dental health care for the patient. Weighing and balancing ethical principles are the major tasks involved in ethical decision making.

■ Principle of Nonmaleficence

The founding principle of all the health professions is *nonmaleficence*. This principle declares that a health care provider's first obligation to the patient is to do no harm (in Latin, *primum non nocere*). Patients place themselves in the care of another person and, at a minimum, should expect that no additional harm will result from that act. The patient grants another person the privilege of access to a portion of his or her body for an explicit purpose, a privilege founded in trust. Fundamental to that trust is that the health care provider will do no harm to the patient.

The Hippocratic Oath requires that the health care provider promise to keep the sick from harm and injustice. In reference to nonmaleficence, the American Dental Association's (ADA) publication, *Principles of Ethics and Code of Professional Conduct,* states that "the principle expresses the concept that professionals have a duty to protect the patient from harm. Under this principle, the dentist's primary obligations include keeping knowledge and skills current, knowing one's own limitations and when to refer to a specialist or other professional, and knowing when and under what circumstances delegation of patient care to auxiliaries is appropriate."[1] For example, practitioners are required to maintain their level of knowledge and skill through participation in appropriate continuing education programs. Thus a dentist who has not performed an endodontic procedure since graduation from dental school 25 years ago would be expected to refer patients to a colleague for root canal therapy. Likewise, a dental hygienist also has an obligation to stay up to date with the changing standards of care in the profession. A hygienist who is unfamiliar with sealant placement procedures or anesthesia techniques should defer performing that service until achieving competency.

Although nonmaleficence primarily is concerned with doing no harm, over time it has evolved to include preventing and removing harm. Therefore health care providers have an obligation to do no harm as well as to prevent harm. Prevention of harm clearly is a domain of dental hygienists. Hygienists are concerned with preventing harm when universal precautions are observed, when scaling and root planing are performed to preserve teeth and periodontal tissues, and when educating patients in home health care. Similarly, dental hygienists remove harm when they treat patients who have active periodontal disease.

Application of Nonmaleficence

Does prevention of harm mean all possible harm? A narrow interpretation of this principle would hold that complete avoidance of any pain and suffering in patient care must be maintained. Such strict interpretation would mean that invasive diagnostic tests to locate disease, as well as intraoral injections to allow scaling and root planing, could never be performed. Consequently patients could never benefit from treatment that would alleviate current pain, and they could not benefit from the prevention of future pain and suffering. This would seem to be an unrealistic application of nonmaleficence. A health care provider may not always be able to avoid harm. In fact, causing some degree of harm when that harm will lead to a greater good—restoring a patient to health—maybe desirable as well as necessary. This conflict is referred to as the *principle of double effect,* and it requires the health care provider to consider the risks and benefits whenever treatment is provided.[2] What comprises harm and good can be delineated by the following classification system[3]:

1 One ought not to inflict harm.
2 One ought to prevent harm.
3 One ought to remove harm.
4 One ought to do or promote good.

The first entry (1) refers to avoidance of harm (nonmaleficence), which takes precedence over the second, third, and fourth entries, which define beneficence, or the promotion of good. This hierarchy of nonmaleficence and beneficence provides the clinician with a guideline to follow in sorting out dilemmas in practice. Not inflicting harm takes precedence over preventing harm, and removing harm is a higher priority than promoting good. Ideally, the dental hygienist would be able to implement all four parts of this hierarchical relationship; however, when faced with constraints and conflict, prioritization would be necessary. Avoiding harm and promoting good in the practice of dental hygiene and dentistry are not always possible.

Principle of Beneficence

Whereas nonmaleficence is concerned with doing no harm to a patient, *beneficence* requires that existing harm be removed. Beneficence focuses on "doing good" for the patient. Doing good requires taking all appropriate actions to restore patients to good health. Health care providers, based on their knowledge and skill, use all reasonable means to benefit the patient. Dentists and hygienists have acquired a body of knowledge and corresponding skills that make them uniquely qualified to help identify patient needs and recommend and provide actions to address those needs. Thus their unique qualifications allow them to benefit the patient by removing existing harm and assisting in the prevention of future harm.

Beneficence and nonmaleficence often are linked because they are both founded in the Hippocratic tradition, which requires the physician to do what will best benefit the patient. This is a consequentialist approach. Meeting the requirement to do what the physician believes will best benefit the patient implies the need to conduct a consequence analysis to determine the best possible outcome for the patient. Beneficence is found in all health care codes. By choosing to become a dental hygienist, an individual assumes a responsibility to help others and professes to be a part of a profession. This means that the hygienist's actions, behaviors, and attitudes must be consistent with a commitment to public service, which is a commitment to benefit others. This commitment to help and benefit others morally defines the healing professions and sets them apart from other occupations, such as architecture or engineering.[4]

Application of Beneficence

For dental hygienists, whose primary focus is preventing oral diseases, promoting good is a daily purpose and goal. Indeed, for any person who is in a position to promote good for the benefit of others, as health care providers are, failure to increase the good of others is morally wrong. The purpose and existence of biomedical research, public health policies and programs, and preventive medicine are the formalized aspects of this part of health care. Society—through various federal, state, and community-based activities—attempts to meet this need for the good of the public. The promotion of good becomes difficult, however, when good is defined according to differing values and belief systems. The teaching of careful oral hygiene self-care to maintain health and function is an example of promotion of good to many people. However, the removal of all carious teeth to eliminate pain and suffering may be considered promoting good to other individuals. In public health programs, the appropriation of limited resources to meet the medical and dental needs of a given population can be a challenging and frustrating exercise but also part of being a health care professional who advocates for the betterment of society.

Principle of Autonomy

Autonomy is self-determination and the ability to be self-governing and self-directing. An autonomous person chooses thoughts and actions relevant to his or her needs, independent from the will of others. In health care autonomy gives rise to the concept of permitting individuals to make decisions about their own health, which is the heart of many ethical dilemmas that occur in dentistry.[5] All health care providers must respect the autonomy of patients and properly inform them about all aspects of the diagnosis, prognosis, and the care being provided. Because dental hygienists have a wide range of knowledge and skills, they must fully and adequately explain the parameters of the services that can be performed as well as the consequences of performing or not performing those services.

Application of Autonomy

The application of autonomy is founded in deontology and is based on respect for persons. The deontologist holds that the health care provider has a duty to allow patients to make decisions about actions that will affect their bodies. The health care provider also has a duty to provide patients with all the unbiased information they would need to make a decision about treatment options. This is an area where potential for conflict exists between what the dentist and/or hygienist believes is in the best interest of the patient and what the patient believes is in his or her best interest. Sometimes what the professional believes is best for the patient is not what the patient elects to do. As long as the patient selects from treatment options that are consistent with accepted standards of care, the professional may ethically act on the patient's choice. However, the professional practitioner also has the autonomy to not provide a service requested by the patient if that service is in conflict with the standards of patient care. For example, refusing a patient's request to extract all healthy teeth would be ethical even though that decision would conflict with the patient's autonomy. Dentists and hygienists will avoid doing harm to a patient even if the patient is exercising autonomy by asking to receive a potentially harmful treatment or service.

Principle of Justice

*A*ll virtue is summed up in dealing justly.

ARISTOTLE

The principle of *justice* is concerned with providing individuals or groups with what is owed, due, or deserved. Nonconsequentialists view justice as a duty for health care providers. The foundation of justice has frequently been described as the principle of equality; likes should be treated alike, equals should be treated as equals, and unequals treated as unequals. The obvious problem in this approach is that some mechanism or criteria must determine who is equal or unequal. If one is unequal, is he or she entitled to the same type and quality of health care as the "equals"? Would that be just? Fundamental to the principle of justice is an effort to treat people who have similar needs in a similar or identical manner. All patients who seek treatment for the prevention of periodontal disease should receive the same level of care and attention from the dental hygienist regardless of personal or social characteristics. For example, consider the case of a large city in the state of Iowa with 3500 people who need the same extensive treatment for periodontal disease. Hypothetically, all have the same oral health needs. Those who have money can, with both professional and home care, save all their teeth. Those without money may lose all their teeth in the next 4 years. Of those who have money, only those who are younger than 60 years are encouraged to participate in complete therapeutic activities to save all their teeth; those who are "foreign" are assumed to not care whether their teeth are saved or lost. Is this just? Regardless of age, gender, social status, religion, or other distinguishing factors, each person should be entitled to the same oral health care options when a similar health care need exists. That would be just.

Justice in dentistry, most often discussed in terms of public policy issues, is further referred to as *distributive justice*. Every society must address the problem of how its resources will be distributed because every society has a scarcity of resources. Resources are scarce whether referring to materials, specially trained individuals, money, or time. **Distributive justice** is concerned with the allocation of resources in large social systems. Policymakers must confront the issue of how society distributes its resources. Who gets what and why? This has implications for national health care policy. Should the United States have a national health care policy? If so, should dentistry be included in any proposed national health care policy? If so, what kind of treatment will be offered, who will provide the treatment, and who will be eligible to receive the treatment?

Justice consists not in being neutral between right and wrong, but in finding out the right and upholding it, wherever found, against the wrong.

THEODORE ROOSEVELT

Application of Justice

If resources were unlimited, the problem of just allocation would be minimal. Unfortunately, that is not the reality of the world in which we live. Choices must be made, benefits and burdens must be balanced, and resources justly distributed. A lofty goal for most organized societies would be the just application of health care. However, no legal mandate exists for medical and dental care to be available to all persons, and decisions are made daily according to the ability of the patient to pay for the services rendered. Thus the provision of dental care is applied unequally. People who present for treatment are, for the most part, granted access to care based on their economic ability and not their dental needs.

The question of who should provide dental care when an economically impoverished individual is in need of treatment is difficult to answer. Many dental hygienists and dentists provide charitable services on a regular basis, either in a private practice office or through participation in a community-based service clinic, because of their recognition of their obligation to serve society. Unfortunately, although this is a lauded practice, it does not come close to meeting the needs of those who cannot access dental care. Many dental public health practitioners and leaders consistently call for the profession to make oral health a much higher priority for federal and state decision makers.

If you tell the truth you don't have to remember anything.

MARK TWAIN

Values and Concepts

Several values and rules support the principles of ethics and add clarity to attempts to make ethical decisions. Many of the concepts are related to the discussion of consequentialism and nonconsequentialism presented in

Chapter 2. Remember that an ethical dilemma occurs when one or more ethical principles are in conflict. Thus values and concepts discussed in this section are founded in ethical principles and the theory upon which those principles are based. Conflict between or among some of these values and concepts is to be expected. They do, however, add clarity to attempts to identify ethical issues and resolve conflicts. These new terms and concepts are paternalism, veracity, informed consent, and confidentiality.

Paternalism

Paternalism arises from the Hippocratic tradition and is closely related to the principles of nonmaleficence and beneficence. The Hippocratic approach is based on the physician (interpreted as including all health care providers in modern times) doing what he or she believes is best for the patient according to his or her ability and judgment. After all, who knows more about oral health and disease than the dentist and hygienist? This approach requires the dentist or hygienist to undertake a role similar to that of a parent. Paternalism means that the health care professional acts as a parent and makes decisions for the patient on the basis of what the professional believes is in the best interest of the patient. Paternalism should never be applied primarily to benefit the professional at the expense of the patient. In fact, many would argue that paternalism should never be applied because it subverts the autonomous wishes of the patient. Thus paternalism and autonomy are in conflict. A dentist or hygienist cannot unilaterally act on behalf of the patient without denying the patient's right to exercise autonomy.

Application of Paternalism.   In general, patients today are well informed about health, treatments, and their rights as patients and want to participate in the decision-making process. In years past, however, paternalism was a common practice partly because the health care provider had superior knowledge and skills and partly because patients expected the health care provider to make decisions in their best interests. Patients often had no knowledge that alternative care options were available. Furthermore, even if patients did know other options existed, many placed the professional in a parental role by asking the professional what they should do. Patients frequently had so much trust in the provider that they would do whatever was suggested. Such paternalistic acts were carried out with good intentions to benefit the patient and often became second nature to the clinician. The historic benchmark for refuting paternalism was a political philosophy essay written in the mid-1800s. Mill's essay remains one of the hallmarks of liberal political theory and is the basis for the societal presumption that individuals are free to act as they see fit.[6]

The responsibility of the dental hygienist is to educate the patient about the balance of benefits and risks of treatment, which often creates a conflict between autonomy and beneficence. This aspect of providing ethical care is most important and requires the dental hygienist to take the time and effort to ensure that the patient has all the knowledge required to make health decisions. A dental hygienist or dentist also can refuse to perform a procedure that he or she considers to not be in the best interest of the patient. Such a decision, which is based on the autonomy of the health care provider, often is done in practice. For example, many dentists have been asked by a patient—and have refused—to remove healthy dentition merely because the patient believes that taking care of dentures would be easier than caring for their natural teeth.

Veracity

> *If* your mouth turns into a knife, it will cut off your lips.
>
> AFRICAN PROVERB

Veracity is defined as being honest and telling the truth. It is the basis of the trust relationship established between a patient and a health care provider. Veracity binds the patient and the clinician as they seek to establish mutual treatment goals. Patients are expected to be truthful about their medical history, treatment expectations, and other relevant facts. Clinicians, for their part, must be truthful about the diagnosis, treatment options, benefits and disadvantages of each treatment option, cost of treatment, and the longevity afforded by the various treatment options. This allows patients to use their autonomy to make decisions in their own best interest. The obligation of veracity, based on respect for patients and autonomy, is acknowledged in most codes of ethics, including the codes of the American Dental Hygienists' Association (ADHA) and the ADA.

Application of Veracity

Lying to a patient does not respect the autonomy of the patient and can compromise any future relationships the patient may have with health care providers. Because relationships are built on trust, lying, even little "white lies," easily erodes trust. *Benevolent deception* is the name given to the practice of withholding information from a patient because of the clinician's belief that the information may harm the individual. This practice is in the tradition of the Hippocratic oath but is not supported by most codes of ethics and then only in extraordinary circumstances. Only a rare case would justify deceit in the dental setting. The interactive health care relationship between patient and clinician functions most effectively when both parties are truthful and adhere to all promises made in the process.

Informed Consent

Informed consent has both ethical and legal implications in medicine and dentistry and is based on the patient exercising autonomy in decision making. Informed consent is two pronged. First, it requires that the professional provide the patient with all relevant information needed to make a decision. Second, it allows the patient to make the decision on the basis of the information provided. Informed consent could be viewed as a process of providing appropriate information to the patient, the process of understanding and assimilating the information, and making the decision. Thus informed consent involves explaining all aspects of health and treatment and ensuring that the patient comprehends what is being explained.

Application of Informed Consent.   As previously noted in the discussion of autonomy, accepting the decision of the patient when it is in conflict with what the health care provider would most highly recommend is extremely difficult for dental professionals. Dentists and hygienists must recognize that the patient has a right to informed consent as well as a right to make an informed refusal. Respecting the autonomy of individuals as self-determining agents recognizes their right to make their own choices and determine their own destiny. This includes the right for a patient to assess all the information provided by the professional yet still make a choice that is not the one most valued by the professional. This is known as *informed refusal.* The media frequently provide details of medical dilemmas when a "wrong" or questionable decision is made for another person. For example, parents in some religious groups refuse to allow life-saving treatments for their sick children or for themselves. Although less dramatic than a life and death decision, dental decisions may involve choices that are potentially harmful to the patient. An example of this was provided in the discussion of the principle of autonomy and obedience to the standards of care.

When patients give their authorization for a procedure or a comprehensive treatment plan, they grant the health care provider informed consent for that treatment. Faden and colleagues[7] state that two kinds of informed consent exist. The first is the set of rules that health care providers must observe to obtain and document information and disclosure; the second is the process of interaction and communication, which produces a truly informed decision.

Not all individuals have the ability to make informed decisions about their dental health. Children and people who are mentally disabled typically have a parent or caregiver who assumes that function. Depending on the age and capacity of the child, certain choices can and should be discussed with the younger patient, but actual decisions regarding what types of services are rendered must remain the purview of the legal guardian. Informed consent when the patient does not understand because of a language barrier is not possible, and steps must be taken to remedy the situation. The use of a translator, family member, or other communication option must be pursued to ensure that the patient fully understands the choices and consequences. To do any less is unethical and illegal. The only exception to this would be if the patient's life were in danger and an immediate procedure were required to save that life.

Confidentiality

Confidentiality is a critical aspect of trust and has a long history of use in the healing arts. Confidentiality is related to respect for persons and involves the patient exercising his or her autonomy in providing information to the professional. The requirement for confidentiality is mentioned in all codes of ethics as well as the Hippocratic oath. Trust is necessary for the exchange of personal and intimate information from the patient to the clinician. A patient has a right to privacy concerning his or her medical and dental history, examination findings, discussion of treatment options and treatment choices, and all records pertaining to dental and dental hygiene care. This privacy extends to the way in which information is gathered, stored, and communicated to other health care professionals. Discussion about a patient's history or treatment is not to be shared with spouses, family, or friends; to do so is a violation of confidentiality. Information about a patient can be given to other health care professionals with the patient's permission. When a case is discussed in an educational setting or a second opinion is sought, the clinician who first saw the patient in question should protect the privacy of the patient.

Application of Confidentiality.   Conflicts and exceptions will arise surrounding the principle of confidentiality. In certain situations legal requirements exist to report diseases that can have an effect on the health of the public, such as sexually transmitted diseases. Reporting suspected child abuse, which is required in most states, is a violation of confidentiality. In dealing with minor children, divulging confidential information to the parents may be necessary to protect the child from harm. This is especially difficult with adolescents, who may or may not be adults according to the legal system. The patient's right to confidentiality often must be balanced against the rights of other individuals. In any situation the health care provider must communicate to the patient the professional and legal responsibilities that exist for disclosure and work toward helping the patient as much as possible.

Fidelity is the belief that it is right to keep promises and fulfill commitments. Some philosophers consider this value as stemming from autonomy and the basic idea of respect for persons. Others denote it as a framework of confidentiality. For the health care provider, it includes the duty to fulfill all portions of *implied* or expressed promises made to the patient in addition to holding to contractual agreements, not abandoning the patient before the completion of treatment, and keeping confidentiality.

> *The secret of the care of the patient is in caring for the patient.*
>
> FRANCIS WELD PEABODY

■ Applying Principles and Values

Basic principles guide the dental hygienist and all health care providers in determining what is right and wrong in the practice of health care. From these principles are derived the rules laid out in all codes of ethics and codes of professional conduct. How these principles and codes are applied to decision making is the challenge for each health care provider faced with a professional problem or dilemma. What does a person do when duties conflict or when more than one principle is involved in a situation?

> *There are two ways of spreading light: to be the candle or the mirror that reflects it.*
>
> EDITH WHARTON

Prima Facie Duties

Thiroux[8] describes *prima facie duties* as duties that must be done before any other considerations enter the picture. Prima facie means "at first glance." He established two rules to deal with the conflict of prima facie duties:

i. Always do the act that is in accord with the stronger prima facie duty.

ii. Always do the act that has the greatest of prima facie rightness over prima facie wrongness.

For example, the dental hygienist who suspects child abuse should place the welfare of the child over the autonomy of the parent. The stronger duty in this instance is the good of the child, not the right of the parent.

These rules, with the supporting principles and values, can provide the dental hygienist guidance in the decision-making process. However, although these are good guides to use, they do not automatically provide correct ethical decisions because they sometimes are in conflict with each other. A choice must be made regarding which rule or value has precedence.

Other Values Used in Health Care

Some textbooks and philosophers may use different approaches to identify principles and values used in health care. Textbooks occasionally classify veracity as one of five major principles rather than as a dimension of autonomy, as defined in this book.[5,9] Codes of ethics also can be developed around concepts that may be structured in a different foundation. The Code of Ethics of the ADHA identifies the following five fundamental principles:

1 Universality
2 Complementarity
3 Ethics
4 Community
5 Responsibility

In addition, it lists the following seven core values on which the standards of professional responsibility are built:

1 Autonomy
2 Confidentiality
3 Trust
4 Nonmaleficence
5 Beneficence
6 Justice
7 Veracity

Universality is a characteristic that states that if two or more people consider the same action or trait in the same situation, the same conclusion would be drawn.[5] That is, if a given situation were duplicated, it would lead to the same evaluative result each time. Complementarity, an aspect of justice that is closely aligned with the consequentialism theory, can be described as doing the greatest good for the greatest number of persons. Discussions about the use and application of public policy resources is an example of complementarity, as is consideration of culture and language in health care services.

The intention in the presentation of principles and values is to provide the precepts that are the underpinnings of a code of ethics or a particular philosophic approach. Whether veracity, confidentiality, and trust are applied according to the four basic principles of nonmaleficence, beneficence, autonomy, and justice or whether an expanded view is adopted, the goal is to identify and apply these guidelines when analyzing an ethical dilemma or pondering a difficult choice between right and wrong.

Summary

This chapter provides an introduction to the fundamental principles of ethics (nonmaleficence, beneficence, autonomy, justice) and several related values and concepts (paternalism, veracity, informed consent, confidentiality) commonly used to assist in ethical decision making. These principles and concepts are intellectual tools that can guide the dental hygienist in making difficult decisions when confronting an ethical dilemma.

REFERENCES

1 Council on Ethics, Bylaws and Judicial Affairs: *Principles of ethics and code of professional conduct*, Chicago, 2008, American Dental Association.
2 Beauchamp TL, Childress J: *Principles of biomedical ethics*, ed 4, New York, 1994, Oxford University Press.
3 Frankena WK: *Ethics*, ed 2, Upper Saddle River, NJ, 1963, Prentice-Hall.
4 Campbell CS, Rodgers VC: The normative principles of dental ethics. In Weinstein BD, ed: *Dental ethics*, Philadelphia, 1993, Lea & Febiger.
5 Rule JT, Veatch RM: *Ethical questions in dentistry*, ed 2, Chicago, 2004, Quintessence.
6 Kahn JP, Hasegawa TK Jr: The dentist-patient relationship. In Weinstein BD, ed: *Dental ethics*, Philadelphia, 1993, Lea & Febiger.
7 Faden RR, King NM, Beauchamp TL: *A history and theory of informed consent*, New York, 1986, Oxford University Press.
8 Thiroux JP: *Ethics theory and practice*, ed 3, New York, 1986, Macmillan.
9 Ozar DT, Sokol DJ: *Dental ethics at chairside: professional principles and practical applications*, ed 2, Washington, DC, 2002, Georgetown University Press.

CHAPTER 4

Social Responsibility and Justice

PHYLLIS L. BEEMSTERBOER
AND FRANK CATALANOTTO

LEARNING OUTCOMES

- Describe the role of the dental hygienist in meeting the oral health care needs of the public.
- Relate the importance of the *Surgeon General's Report on Oral Health* to the profession of dental hygiene.
- Describe the issue of access to care and social responsibility.
- Identify several strategies that a dental hygienist can implement in striving for social justice.

KEY TERMS

access to care
health disparities

social contract
social justice

The dental hygienist assumes the rights and responsibilities of service in the greater good as a health care provider and a professional. This chapter reviews the issues of disparity in oral health care, **access to care,** and the responsibilities of all oral health care professionals to advocate just distribution of resources to meet the oral health care needs of the public.

If you haven't any charity in your heart, you have the worst kind of heart trouble.

BOB HOPE

Disparities in Oral Health Care

Surgeon General's Report on Oral Health

The first *Surgeon General's Report on Oral Health* was published in 2000. This landmark report described the meaning of oral health and explained why oral health is essential to general health and well-being.[1] After the publication of more than 50 surgeon general reports, to have one specifically on oral health was a major event and highlighted how much progress had been made in understanding common oral diseases. The use of "oral health" and not "dental health" was a deliberate choice of words because oral health means more than healthy teeth. The report included conditions and diseases such as oral cancers, lesions of the head and neck, birth defects, and facial pain. The phase "the mouth is a mirror" of the body was used to emphasize the relation of mouth to body and to point to the association of oral-systemic disease connections. The report established that oral health is integral to general health and that the two should not be looked at separately. Oral health is a critical component of overall health.

The surgeon general's report also addressed the disparities and inequalities that affect the most vulnerable populations: the poor, children, the elderly, the disabled, and racial and ethnic minorities. These groups often cannot access care for financial reasons, but lack of access also can be caused by fear and complex psychosocial or cultural assumptions. How to address this need is a social responsibility of all health care professionals working with public and private agencies. It a complex and challenging problem in which the dental hygienist is well suited to be an active participant.

MAJOR FINDINGS OF ORAL HEALTH IN AMERICA

- Oral diseases and disorders affect health and well-being throughout life.
- Safe and effective measures exist to prevent common oral diseases.
- The mouth reflects general health and well-being.
- Oral diseases and conditions are associated with other health problems.
- Lifestyle behaviors that affect general health affect oral and craniofacial health.
- Profound and consequential oral health disparities are present in the U.S. population.
- More information is needed to improve oral health and eliminate health disparities.
- Research is the key to further reduction in the burden of diseases and disorders that affect the craniofacial complex.

Data from U.S. Department of Health and Human Services: Oral health in America: a report of the surgeon general, *Rockville, Md, 2000, National Institutes of Health.*

*W*hat we must decide is perhaps how we are valuable, rather than how valuable we are.

F. SCOTT FITZGERALD

National Institutes of Health Report on Oral Health Disparities

The National Institute of Dental and Craniofacial Research continued to examine the disparity issue by publishing *A Plan to Eliminate Craniofacial, Oral and Dental Health Disparities* in 2002.[2] This report listed many factors besides finances that must be identified when determining why certain populations become patients and others do not. By 2050 racial and ethnic minority groups are expected to no longer be "minorities" but will constitute the emerging majority of the U.S. population. Social, political, economic, and cultural factors clearly underlie the complex social problem of inequality. Although these problems are not new, they continue to confound and frustrate. The deaths of two children from dental abscesses made headlines in 2006 and triggered some legislative actions that may begin to prevent this kind of tragedy.[3]

Health Disparities and Professionalism

As a society, we are faced with disparities in health care and in dental health care. More than 47 million people in the United States are estimated to be underinsured or have no health insurance; this is a great concern for the public health and well-being of the country.[4,5] An even larger percentage of the population does not have dental insurance or has minimal dental benefits. Dental hygienists are focused on prevention, a focus that fits well with the goals of health promotion that have been established by the U.S. Department of Health and Human Services. Over the years the surgeon general of the Public Health Service has focused attention on important public health issues. Formal reports of the surgeon general on the adverse health consequences of smoking began and continue nationwide efforts to prevent tobacco use. Other reports on topics such as nutrition, youth violence, bone health, mental health, and HIV/AIDS have provided information and awareness of important public health issues. Most of these reports have generated major public health initiatives and eventual changes in health approaches and practices.

> **W**herever there is a human being, there is an opportunity for kindness.
>
> LUCIUS SENECA

The responsibility of all oral health care professionals to assist and lead society in finding solutions to oral **health disparities** is based on the historic definition of a profession.[6] This concept of service and the aspirations for professionalism in dental hygiene are established in the code of ethics and addressed in its fundamental principles and core values. Listed under *Standards of Professional Responsibility, Community, and Society* are several points that include increasing access to care, promoting public health, supporting justice, and recognizing an obligation to provide pro bono service. As a group dental hygienists aspire to make a contribution to the public and to enhance for all the ability to seek and receive dental care resources. Dental care is, by its nature, a social enterprise even when normally provided on a one-on-one basis.[7] The **social contract** made between the public and health care professionals, such as dental hygienists and dentists, is the basis of this relationship.

Dental hygienists and dentists take pride in being recognized as professional health care providers. Welie,[8-10] in a series of articles examining what it means to be a professional, defined a profession as a "collective of expert services providers who have jointly and publicly committed to always give priority to the existential needs and interests of the public they serve above their own and who in turn are trusted by the public to do so." Thus the benefit of being called a professional also carries the burden of addressing the needs of the public. How the dental hygienist uses his or her skills and knowledge to advance the public good is part of the obligation laid out in the code of ethics and embraced in the essence of a professional person. We must consider our obligations as a group, not just individuals who are members of a group, by honoring the justice principle in the code of ethics and sharing ethical concerns as a moral community.[11,12]

Ethical Goals in Oral Health Care

The values of caring, stewardship, and justice are of great importance for achieving ethical goals in health care, the goals that focus on society. These are different from the ethical principles that focus on the individual, such as autonomy and self-determination. Justice in dental care is a complex topic. What is just or fair? What does the just distribution of dental health care resources look like? For the parents of a child with a toothache who can find a dentist and pay for dental services, no dilemma exists. For the parents of a child with a toothache who cannot find a dentist because they have no ability to pay for services or have no access to a public program, a dilemma certainly exists, as does the need to examine the disparities of the situation. As discussed in Chapter 3, *distributive justice* is the term used when discussing allocation of resources in large social systems. Saying that everyone should have access to dental care is easy; but what kind of care are individuals entitled to when resources are limited? The first response might be basic dental care or adequate dental care. Defining what that might be is a daunting task that challenges communities and the federal government. Even the term *access* can be misleading, with access defined as a freedom or ability to obtain, and *accessibility* defined as the ease with which health care can be reached in the face of barriers such as finance or culture.[13] As Garetto and Yoder[14] stated, we also have a responsibility to those who are unaware of need, do not seek it, cannot get to it, or are afraid of it. Ethically, the goal of improving the health of the population is a societal greater good benefiting society at large.

> *The best way to find yourself is to lose yourself in the service of others.*
>
> MAHATMA GANDHI

Social Justice

Numerous authors and national reports have addressed the importance of teaching social responsibility as part of professionalism. Two Institute of Medicine reports in the early 2000s advocated increased professionalism and **social justice** as a part of improving quality and bridging the gaps in health care.[15,16] The American Dental Education Association defined its role and responsibility with its member institutions in improving the oral health status of all Americans in a report in 2003.[17] The findings stressed the importance of increasing the diversity of the oral health workforce and teaching and exhibiting values that prepare future dental professionals to commit to delivering oral health care to all populations, including the underserved. The message from the health care professions is that professionalism includes social responsibility, an ethic of caring and access to that care for all members of society.[18]

AMERICAN DENTAL EDUCATION ASSOCIATION RECOMMENDATIONS FOR IMPROVING THE ORAL HEALTH STATUS OF ALL AMERICANS

Roles and Responsibilities of Academic Dental Institutions
- Monitor future oral health care workforce needs.
- Improve the effectiveness of the oral health care delivery system.
- Prepare students to provide oral health services to diverse populations.
- Increase the diversity of the oral health workforce.
- Improve the effectiveness of allied dental professionals in reaching the underserved.

Data from Haden NK, Catalanotto FA, Alexander CJ, et al: Improving the oral health status of all Americans: roles and responsibilities of academic dental institutions: the report of the ADEA President's Commission, J Dent Educ 67:563, 2003.

Role of the Dental Hygienist

Most dental hygienists work in an employer/employee setting where a solo dentist or small group of dentists owns and runs the dental care business. It is not prudent or feasible for an employee in such a situation to provide free or discounted dental hygiene care; this kind of "band-aid" approach would not solve the greater problem anyway.[19,20] However, the dental hygienist can be a part of the movement to alleviate disparities and develop effective care systems in many ways.

Following are some suggested activities to address these societal disparities:

- Provide dental hygiene services at a safety net clinic.
- Work on a community campaign to install fluoridation in the local water district.
- Participate in state-organized caries prevention programs.
- Work with local dental groups to address oral health disparities.
- Support school-based fluoride and sealant programs.
- Volunteer at general and dental health fairs.
- Provide dental hygiene services in mobile dental vans.
- Support collaborations among community-based programs and practitioners.
- Educate patients regarding the importance of public programs and dental health.
- Educate local, state, and federal policymakers on access to care issues.
- Become involved in discussions regarding public health infrastructure.
- Support research on oral health and disparities.
- Recruit individuals to join the oral health workforce.
- Keep informed on care delivery systems, reimbursement schedules, and changes in public policy.
- Advocate improved funding and access for Medicaid recipients.
- Advocate better dental insurance and the inclusion of dental benefits in any new national health insurance plans.
- Advocate increased scope of practice regulations, or new workforce models, at the state or national level that would allow dental hygienists to provide more care to underserved patients in a variety of settings.

Summary

Improving oral health care can take many avenues in which the dental hygienist can be an active and effective participant. The dental hygienist, along with other health care providers, must recognize the collective and individual responsibilities held as health professionals to address the oral health needs of the entire public. Collaboration among many stakeholders in providing access to dental care is part of being a professional and caring member of society.

The test of our progress is not whether we add more to the abundance of those who have much; it is whether we provide enough for those who have too little.

FRANKLIN D. ROOSEVELT

REFERENCES

1 U.S. Department of Health and Human Services: *Oral health in America: a report of the surgeon general,* Rockville, Md, 2000, National Institutes of Health.

2 U.S. Department of Health and Human Services: *A plan to eliminate craniofacial, oral and dental health disparities,* Rockville, Md, 2002, National Institutes of Health.

3 Otto M: For want of a dentist, *Washington Post,* February 28, 2007.

4 Edelstein BL: Disparities in oral health and access to care: findings of national surveys, *Ambulatory Pediatrics* 2(2 suppl):141, 2002.

5 Garcia RI: Addressing oral health disparities in diverse populations, *J Am Dent Assoc* 136:1210, 2005.

6 Pellegrino ED: What is a profession, *J Appl Health* 12(3):168, 1983.

7 Ozar DT, Sokol DJ: *Dental ethics at chairside: professional principles and practical applications,* ed 2, Washington, 2002, Georgetown University Press.

8 Welie JVM: Is dentistry a profession? Part I: professionalism defined, *J Can Dent Assoc* 70(8):529, 2004.

9 Welie JVM: Is dentistry a profession? Part II: hallmarks of professionalism, *J Can Dent Assoc* 70(9):599, 2004.

10 Welie JVM: Is dentistry a profession? Part III: future challenges, *J Can Dent Assoc* 70(10):675, 2004.

11 Dharamsi S, MacEntee M: Dentistry and distributive justice, *Soc Sci Med* 55:323, 2002.

12 Dharamsi S: Building moral communities? First, do no harm, *J Dent Educ* 70(11):1235, 2006.

13 Crall JJ: Access to oral health care: professional and societal considerations, *J Dent Educ* 70(11):1133, 2006.

14 Garetto LP, Yoder KM: Basic oral health needs: a professional priority? *J Dent Educ* 70(11):1166, 2006.

15 Institute of Medicine: *Crossing the quality chasm: a new health system for the 21st century,* Washington, DC, 2001, National Academies Press.

16 Institute of Medicine: *Health professions education: a bridge to quality,* Washington, DC, 2003, National Academies Press.

17 Haden NK, Catalanotto FA, Alexander CJ, et al: Improving the oral health status of all Americans: roles and responsibilities of academic dental institutions: the report of the ADEA President's Commission, *J Dent Educ* 67:563, 2003.

18 Beemsterboer PL: Developing an ethic of access to care in dentistry, *J Dent Educ* 70(11):1212, 2006.

19 Mouradian WE: Band-Aid solutions to the dental access crisis: conceptually flawed—a response, *J Dent Educ* 70(11):1174, 2006.

20 U.S. Department of Health and Human Services: *National healthcare quality report,* Rockville, Md, 2005, National Institutes of Health.

CHAPTER 5

Codes of Ethics

PHYLLIS L. BEEMSTERBOER

LEARNING OUTCOMES

- Discuss the role of a code of ethics for the health care professions.
- Explain the value to the public of a professional code of ethics.
- Describe how a code of ethics can assist in the professional duty of self-regulation.
- Compare the 1927 version and the current version of the *Code of Ethics for Dental Hygienists.*
- List and describe the nine sections identified under the *Standards of Professional Responsibilities of the Code of Ethics for Dental Hygienists.*
- Be familiar with the code of the American Dental Association.

KEY TERMS

code of ethics

Hippocratic oath

obligation

professional autonomy

professional code

A *code of ethics* is one of the essential characteristics of a true profession. It is a guideline for members of a professional group used for self-regulation of the group. A major purpose of a *professional code* of ethics is to bind the members of a group together by expressing their goals and aspirations, as well as define expected standards of behavior. The code is the contract the profession makes with society outlining the standards it will adhere to and uphold.

> Knowing is not enough; we must apply. Willing is not enough; we must do.
>
> GOETHE

Professional Codes in Health Care

Ethical codes address the areas of personal integrity, dedication, and principled behavior.[1] Most health care providers cherish and hold sacred the obligations that flow from entrance into a profession. Acceptance and support of the prescribed principles and standards of behavior help reinforce the significance of being a part of a special group of people who are committed to the same values and goals.

Both professional groups and the public have sometimes questioned the value of codes of ethics. Do codes of ethics really make a difference in the way health care providers interact with and treat patients and colleagues? If a member of a profession has seen evidence of colleagues acting unethically and those colleagues have not been punished, that question is legitimate. It would be the same for a member of the public who has had a bad experience with a health care provider. The patient may assume that he or she was treated in a manner inconsistent with the standards of behavior in the profession (even though the professional may have behaved appropriately). Sometimes the act may be inappropriate behavior by the professional; conversely, the frustration of the patient may lead him or her to believe unethical behavior occurred even when it has not.

How, then, does a person know whether codes of ethics are ever effective? Three things demonstrate how codes can be effective in shaping professional behavior. First, when professional schools of health care screen applicants for admission to education programs, integrity and character are important criteria for acceptance. Admissions committees aim to select candidates who are the best qualified academically as well as candidates of good character. Virtue ethics, derived from the tradition of Plato and Aristotle, was introduced in Chapter 2. Virtue is a character trait; the assumption is that if a person is virtuous he or she will act virtuously. Thus part of the selection process focuses on identifying virtue in the character of applicants.

Second, until proven otherwise, each entering student must be assumed to have the character traits needed to be true professional. Educational institutions actively seek to indoctrinate students to the goals of the profession and expected professional behaviors. Learning what is expected of that professional person reinforces character traits in the developing professional. This often is accomplished by introducing students to the institution's code of conduct, by familiarizing them with the profession's code of ethics and professional conduct, by faculty serving as positive role models, and by enforcing adherence to expected professional behaviors when professional codes have been violated.

Third, after entering professional practice, it becomes the **obligation** of those professionals to help regulate their profession. When violations occur, members of the profession who become aware of these violations have a duty to intervene in a substantive way. This is a serious step and must be carefully considered; the reputation of the profession and the well-being of the public ultimately rest on a willingness to engage in meaningful self-policing of the profession.

The degree to which codes are effective remains a difficult question to answer completely. However, because health professions invest so much effort in the development and propagation of codes of ethics and standards of professional behavior, an assumption that the professions find them to be extremely valuable is reasonable. When violations of the code occur, the profession is empowered to take action to resolve the problem. Although codes alone do not guarantee that everyone will behave with integrity, they do provide guidance and standards by which professionals can be judged. Codes also serve as a touchstone by which all members of a profession can judge the acceptable parameters of behavior. This is why being a professional person is a privilege and carries both benefits and responsibilities.

Always do right. This will gratify some people, and astonish the rest.

MARK TWAIN

▪ Development of Ethical Codes

The first ethical code dates back to the time of the Greek physician Hippocrates, and the influence of the *Hippocratic oath* is still reflected today in modern versions of ethical codes (Box 5-1). Traditional medical codes of

---

BOX 5-1

Hippocratic Oath

I swear by Apollo Physician and Asclepios and Hygeia and Panacea and all the gods and goddesses, making them my witnesses, that I will fulfill according to my ability and judgment this oath and this covenant:

To hold him who has taught me this art as equal to my parents and to live my life in partnership with him, and if he is in need of money to give him a share of mine, and to regard his offspring as equal to my brothers in male lineage and to teach them this art—if they desire to learn it—without fee and covenant; to give a share of precepts and oral instruction and all the other learning to my sons and to the sons of him who has instructed me and to pupils who have signed the covenant and have taken an oath according to the medical law, but no one else.

I will apply dietetic measures for the benefit of the sick according to my ability and judgment; I will keep them from harm and injustice.

I will neither give a deadly drug to anybody who asked for it, nor will I make a suggestion to this effect. Similarly I will not give to a woman an abortive remedy. In purity and holiness I will guard my life and my art.

I will not use the knife, not even on sufferers from stone, but will withdraw in favor of such men as are engaged in this work.

Whatever houses I may visit, I will come for the benefit of the sick, remaining free of all intentional injustice, of all mischief and in particular of sexual relations with both female and male persons, be they free or slaves.

What I may see or hear in the course of the treatment or even outside of the treatment in regard to the life of men, which on no account one must spread abroad, I will keep to myself, holding such things shameful to be spoken about.

If I fulfill this oath and do not violate it, may it be granted to me to enjoy life and art, being honored with fame among all men for all time to come; if I transgress it and swear falsely, may the opposite of all this be my lot.

ethics emphasize the physician's (1) duties in the individual patient-physician relationship, including the obligation of confidentiality; (2) authority and duty of beneficence (i.e., acting for the patient's good); and (3) obligation to each other.[2] In return for the power and prestige granted to the professions, a code of ethics is the promise to society to uphold certain values and standards in the practice of the profession. As previously noted, codes of ethics are aspirational in nature. They typically are powerful ethical statements, but they are not legal mandates. However, codes cannot easily be dismissed if there is a formal structure for self-regulation. In recent years evidence is increasing that state dental boards, which usually have authority over both dentists and dental hygienists, are sanctioning practitioners for legal violations as well as ethical violations. Because these boards typically have the authority to suspend or terminate a professional's right to practice, the fact that more attention is being given to ethical behavior makes the relation between ethical codes and enforcement stronger. Ideally, codes should create a relationship among members of a profession that is similar to the ties in a family, obviating the need for enforcement outside the group. Professionals' obligations to each other, to patients, and to society should be similar to the strong obligations and emotional feelings that attend belonging to a family, with the behavior of members being monitored by the membership.

A sound and deep understanding of the moral responsibilities of those entrusted with the health of others is essential.[3] Health care providers have a special responsibility to the patients they treat because of their knowledge and the dependency of the patient on that knowledge. A code of ethics also is a set of commandments and, as such, has two principle functions. First, it provides an enforceable standard of minimally decent conduct for those who fall below that standard. Second, it indicates in general terms some of the ethical considerations a professional must consider when deciding on conduct.[4] The code of ethics can and does serve as a tool in the function of self-regulation.

The use of professional codes in health care has some limitations. Not every situation can be addressed in an ethical code or fully explained in an accompanying interpretation. Some philosophers have noted that most codes stress the obligations of health care professionals rather than describe the rights of those receiving health care services.[5] The current use of a patient's bill of rights in health care settings is an attempt to address this discrepancy.

Intelligence plus character is the goal of a true education.

MARTIN LUTHER KING, JR.

■ Ethical Code for Dental Hygiene

The first code of ethics for dental hygienists was created at the inception of the American Dental Hygienists' Association (ADHA) in 1927.[6] That code, developed in three sections that list the duties of the profession to patients, reads as follows:

> **Section 1:** The dental hygienist should be ever ready to respond to the wants of her patrons, and should fully recognize the obligations involved in the discharge of her duties toward them. As she is in most cases unable to correctly estimate the character of her operations, her own sense of right must guarantee faithfulness in their performance. Her manner should be firm, yet kind and sympathizing so as to gain the respect and confidence of her patients, and even the simplest case committed to her care should receive that attention which is due to operations performed on living, sensitive tissue.
>
> **Section 2:** It is not to be expected that the patient will possess a very extended or very accurate knowledge of professional matters. The dental hygienist should make due allowance for this, patiently explaining many things which seem quite clear to herself, thus endeavoring to educate the public mind so that it will properly appreciate the beneficent efforts of our profession. She should encourage no false hopes by promising success when in the nature of the case there is uncertainty.
>
> **Section 3:** The dental hygienist should be temperate in all things, keeping both mind and body in the best possible health, that her patients may have the benefit of the clearness of judgment and skill which is their right.

The wording of the original code reflects the tone and verbiage of the time and the fact that initially only women were dental hygienists. The code has been revised several times over the years, most significantly in 1995 after a thoughtful review and the incorporation of newer aspects of health care and changes in the profession. Minor revisions have been undertaken in more recent years. This version of the code is presented in several sections and encompasses the areas of endeavor in which the dental hygienist functions. The four goals of the code of ethics are listed in the beginning of the code, and these capture the essence of why the code is important to dental hygienists and the public who entrust themselves for care and services. The key concepts, basic beliefs, fundamental principles, and core values are established and explained in the code so that the standards of professional responsibility can be fully understood by professional and public alike. For dental hygiene students, the code of ethics for dental hygienists is a vehicle for educating novices about the obligations of the profession, informing them about the basic beliefs and fundamental principles of the group, and providing guidelines regarding the expected behavior of a dental hygiene practitioner.

All professional codes are evolving documents that embody the contract between a particular profession and the public. For dental hygiene, the code is maintained by the professional organization (the ADHA) and is monitored by the executive staff of the organization. When deemed necessary, the officers of the association appoint a committee of members to review and revise the document. The code can be amended at any meeting of the ADHA House of Delegates by a two-thirds vote of that group. ADHA and all health care professional organizations have, as a condition of membership, an agreement to uphold the profession's code of ethics.

The code of ethics that was first developed in 1995 is more comprehensive than earlier versions and provides extensive guidance for the dental hygienist working in a variety of health care delivery settings. The current code lists the core principles embraced and upheld in all health care professions and clearly defines for all the standards of professional responsibility that the ADHA believes its members should adhere to in the performance of their services. A code of ethics is a reference and a guide. It should be studied by students and referred to for guidance by working professionals. The ADHA *Code of Ethics for Dental Hygienists* is presented in Appendix 5-1 at the end of this chapter (Figure 5-1).

As I am the younger and not so experienced, I think that I ought certainly to hear first what my elders have to say, and to learn of them, and if I have anything to add, then I may venture to give my opinion and advice to them as well as to you.

SOCRATES

Dental Code

The code for dentists is embodied in the *Principles of Ethics and Code of Professional Conduct* of the American Dental Association (ADA). The code is maintained and updated by the association through its Council of Ethics, Bylaws, and Judicial Affairs. The ADA code is divided into three components: principles of ethics, code of professional conduct, and advisory opinions. The principles of ethics component sets out the aspirational goals of the dental

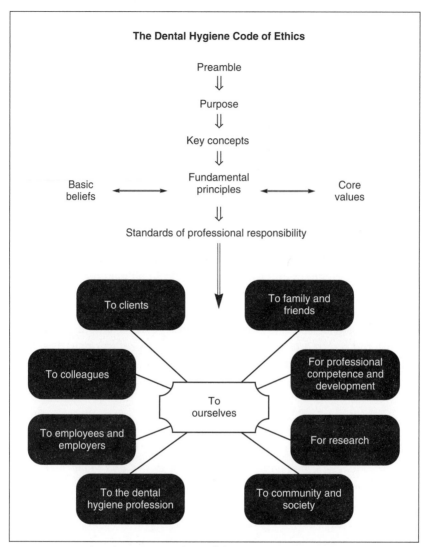

FIGURE 5-1   Visual representation of the American Dental Hygienists'
Association *Dental Hygiene Code of Ethics.* **Although the specific language**
of the code has been updated through the years, its basic components and
aims remain the same. (From American Dental Hygienists' Association: *The dental hygiene code*
of ethics, Chicago, 1995, Author, as appeared in the January 1995 issue of *Access* magazine. Reproduced with
permission of American Dental Hygienists' Association in the format Textbook via Copyright Clearance Center.)

profession, which are similar to the aspirational goals for the dental hygiene
profession. However, the ADA code refers to five fundamental principles,
whereas the ADHA code identifies seven core values, adding confidentiality

TABLE 5-1

Comparison of Principles between ADHA and ADA Codes of Ethics

ADHA CODE	ADA CODE
Individual autonomy	Autonomy
Beneficence	Beneficence
Nonmaleficence	Nonmaleficence
Justice and fairness	Justice
Veracity	Veracity
Confidentiality	
Societal trust	

and societal trust as essential to the foundation of the code. The portion of the ADA code that addresses conduct for dentists—the code of professional conduct—delineates conduct that is either required or prohibited. Each section of the code of professional conduct is followed by an advisory opinion. These opinions expand on an issue and often include legal warnings or suggestions for the dentist to seek further information or advice. Guidance is provided in the ADA code for anyone who believes a member dentist has acted unethically, and the code further explains that censure or suspension can result from a fair hearing on any unethical conduct. The ADA code, with official advisory opinions revised in late 2008, is provided for reference in Appendix A.

The dental hygienist is most often an employee of a dentist. Individuals employed by a dentist should be familiar with the ADA code as well as the ADHA code. A comparison of the principles in both codes is provided in Table 5-1.

Ability is what you're capable of doing. Motivation determines what you do. Attitude determines how well you do it.

LOU HOLTZ

Summary

Codes of ethics are the written standards to which health care professionals agree to adhere before society, which grants certain privileges to these groups. Among these privileges is societal trust and self-regulation. Once an individual has gained the necessary professional knowledge and skill and acquired a professional license, which is an acknowledgment of this achievement, he or she is accorded professional status. The responsibility that goes with this status is to uphold the core values of the profession of dental hygiene: *professional autonomy,* confidentiality, societal trust, non-maleficence, beneficence, justice, and veracity.

REFERENCES

1 Edge RS, Groves JR: *Ethics of health care,* ed 2, New York, 1999, Delmar, p 84.
2 Kenny NP: Codes and character: the pillars of professional ethics, *J Am Coll Dent* 65(3):5, 1998.
3 Jonsen AR: The sins of specialists, *J Hist Dent* 55(3):113, 2007.
4 Benjamin M, Curtis J: *Ethics in nursing,* ed 2, New York, 1986, Oxford University Press, p 6.
5 Beauchamp TL, Childress JF: *Principles of biomedical ethics,* ed 4, New York, 1994, Oxford University Press.
6 Steele PF: *Dimensions of dental hygiene,* ed 3, Philadelphia, 1982, Lea & Febiger, p 474.

APPENDIX 5-1

American Dental Hygienists' Association *Code of Ethics for Dental Hygienists*

1 Preamble

As dental hygienists, we are a community of professionals devoted to the prevention of disease and the promotion and improvement of the public's health. We are preventive oral health professionals who provide educational, clinical, and therapeutic services to the public. We strive to live meaningful, productive, satisfying lives that simultaneously serve us, our profession, our society, and the world. Our actions, behaviors, and attitudes are consistent with our commitment to public service. We endorse and incorporate the Code into our daily lives.

2 Purpose

The purpose of a professional code of ethics is to achieve high levels of ethical consciousness, decision making, and practice by the members of the profession. Specific objectives of the Dental Hygiene Code of Ethics are:

- to increase our professional and ethical consciousness and sense of ethical responsibility.
- to lead us to recognize ethical issues and choices and to guide us in making more informed ethical decisions.
- to establish a standard for professional judgment and conduct.
- to provide a statement of the ethical behavior the public can expect from us.

From American Dental Hygienists' Association: *Code of ethics for dental hygienists*, Chicago, 2007-2008, Author.

The Dental Hygiene Code of Ethics is meant to influence us throughout our careers. It stimulates our continuing study of ethical issues and challenges us to explore our ethical responsibilities. The Code establishes concise standards of behavior to guide the public's expectations of our profession and supports dental hygiene practice, laws and regulations. By holding ourselves accountable to meeting the standards stated in the Code, we enhance the public's trust on which our professional privilege and status are founded.

3 Key Concepts

Our beliefs, principles, values, and ethics are concepts reflected in the Code. They are the essential elements of our comprehensive and definitive code of ethics and are interrelated and mutually dependent.

4 Basic Beliefs

We recognize the importance of the following beliefs that guide our practice and provide context for our ethics:

- The services we provide contribute to the health and well-being of society.
- Our education and licensure qualify us to serve the public by preventing and treating oral disease and helping individuals achieve and maintain optimal health.
- Individuals have intrinsic worth, are responsible for their own health, and are entitled to make choices regarding their health.
- Dental hygiene care is an essential component of overall health care, and we function interdependently with other health care providers.
- All people should have access to health care, including oral health care.
- We are individually responsible for our actions and the quality of care we provide.

5 Fundamental Principles

These fundamental principles, universal concepts, and general laws of conduct provide the foundation for our ethics.

From American Dental Hygienists' Association: *Code of ethics for dental hygienists,* Chicago, 2007-2008, Author.

Universality

The principle of universality expects that, if one individual judges an action to be right or wrong in a given situation, other people considering the same action in the same situation would make the same judgment.

Complementarity

The principle of complementarity recognizes the existence of an obligation to justice and basic human rights. In all relationships, it requires considering the values and perspectives of others before making decisions or taking actions affecting them.

Ethics

Ethics are the general standards of right and wrong that guide behavior within society. As generally accepted actions, they can be judged by determining the extent to which they promote good and minimize harm. Ethics compel us to engage in health promotion/disease prevention activities.

Community

This principle expresses our concern for the bond between individuals, the community, and society in general. It leads us to preserve natural resources and inspires us to show concern for the global environment.

Responsibility

Responsibility is central to our ethics. We recognize that there are guidelines for making ethical choices and accept responsibility for knowing and applying them. We accept the consequences of our actions or the failure to act and are willing to make ethical choices and publicly affirm them.

▪ 6 Core Values

We acknowledge these values as general for our choices and actions.

Individual Autonomy and Respect for Human Beings

People have the right to be treated with respect. They have the right to informed consent prior to treatment, and they have the right to full disclosure of all relevant information so that they can make informed choices about their care.

Confidentiality

We respect the confidentiality of client information and relationships as a demonstration of the value we place on individual autonomy. We acknowledge our obligation to justify any violation of a confidence.

Societal Trust

We value client trust and understand that public trust in our profession is based on our actions and behavior.

Nonmaleficence

We accept our fundamental obligation to provide services in a manner that protects all clients and minimizes harm to them and others involved in their treatment.

Beneficence

We have a primary role in promoting the well being of individuals and the public by engaging in health promotion/disease prevention activities.

Justice and Fairness

We value justice and support the fair and equitable distribution of health care resources. We believe all people should have access to high-quality, affordable oral health care.

Veracity

We accept our obligation to tell the truth and expect that others will do the same. We value self-knowledge and seek truth and honesty in all relationships.

7 Standards of Professional Responsibility

We are obligated to practice our profession in a manner that supports our purpose, beliefs, and values in accordance with the fundamental principles that support our ethics. We acknowledge the following responsibilities:

From American Dental Hygienists' Association: *Code of ethics for dental hygienists*, Chicago, 2007-2008, Author.

To Ourselves as Individuals. . .

- Avoid self-deception and continually strive for knowledge and personal growth.
- Establish and maintain a lifestyle that supports optimal health.
- Create a safe work environment.
- Assert our own interests in ways that are fair and equitable.
- Seek the advice and counsel of others when challenged with ethical dilemmas.
- Have realistic expectations of ourselves and recognize our limitations.

To Ourselves as Professionals. . .

- Enhance professional competencies through continuous learning in order to practice according to high standards of care.
- Support dental hygiene peer-review systems and quality-assurance measures.
- Develop collaborative professional relationships and exchange knowledge to enhance our own lifelong professional development.

To Family and Friends. . .

- Support the efforts of others to establish and maintain healthy lifestyles and respect the rights of friends and family.

To Clients. . .

- Provide oral health care utilizing high levels of professional knowledge, judgment, and skill.
- Maintain a work environment that minimizes the risk of harm.
- Serve all clients without discrimination and avoid action toward any individual or group that may be interpreted as discriminatory.
- Hold professional client relationships confidential.
- Communicate with clients in a respectful manner.
- Promote ethical behavior and high standards of care by all dental hygienists.
- Serve as an advocate for the welfare of clients.
- Provide clients with the information necessary to make informed decisions about their oral health and encourage their full participation in treatment decisions and goals.

- Refer clients to other health care providers when their needs are beyond our ability or scope of practice.
- Educate clients about high-quality oral health care.

To Colleagues. . .

- Conduct professional activities and programs, and develop relationships in ways that are honest, responsible, and appropriately open and candid.
- Encourage a work environment that promotes individual professional growth and development.
- Collaborate with others to create a work environment that minimizes risk to the personal health and safety of our colleagues.
- Manage conflicts constructively.
- Support the efforts of other dental hygienists to communicate the dental hygiene philosophy and preventive oral care.
- Inform other health care professionals about the relationship between general and oral health.
- Promote human relationships that are mutually beneficial, including those with other health care professionals.

To Employees and Employers. . .

- Conduct professional activities and programs and develop relationships in ways that are honest, responsible, open, and candid.
- Manage conflicts constructively.
- Support the right of our employees and employers to work in an environment that promotes wellness.
- Respect the employment rights of our employers and employees.

To the Dental Hygiene Profession. . .

- Participate in the development and advancement of our profession.
- Avoid conflicts of interest and declare them when they occur.
- Seek opportunities to increase public awareness and understanding of oral health practices.

From American Dental Hygienists' Association: *Code of ethics for dental hygienists,* Chicago, 2007-2008, Author.

- Act in ways that bring credit to our profession while demonstrating appropriate respect for colleagues in other professions.
- Contribute time, talent, and financial resources to support and promote our profession.
- Promote a positive image for our profession.
- Promote a framework for professional education that develops dental hygiene competencies to meet the oral and overall health needs of the public.

To the Community and Society...

- Recognize and uphold the laws and regulations governing our profession.
- Document and report inappropriate, inadequate, or substandard care and/or illegal activities by a health care provider, to the responsible authorities.
- Use peer review as a mechanism for identifying inappropriate, inadequate, or substandard care provided by dental hygienists.
- Comply with local, state, and federal statutes that promote public health and safety.
- Develop support systems and quality-assurance programs in the workplace to assist dental hygienists in providing the appropriate **standard of care.**
- Promote access to dental hygiene services for all, supporting justice and fairness in the distribution of health care resources.
- Act consistently with the ethics of the global scientific community of which our profession is a part.
- Create a healthful workplace ecosystem to support a healthy environment.
- Recognize and uphold our obligation to provide pro bono service.

To Scientific Investigation...

We accept responsibility for conducting research according to the fundamental principles underlying our ethical beliefs in compliance with universal codes, governmental standards, and professional guidelines for the care and management of experimental subjects. We acknowledge our ethical obligations to the scientific community:

- Conduct research that contributes knowledge that is valid and useful to our clients and society.

- Use research methods that meet accepted scientific standards.
- Use research resources appropriately.
- Systematically review and justify research in progress to insure the most favorable benefit-to-risk ratio to research subjects.
- Submit all proposals involving human subjects to an appropriate human subject review committee.
- Secure appropriate institutional committee approval for the conduct of research involving animals.
- Obtain informed consent from human subjects participating in research that is based on specification published in Title 21 Code of Federal Regulations Part 46.
- Respect the confidentiality and privacy of data.
- Seek opportunities to advance dental hygiene knowledge through research by providing financial, human, and technical resources whenever possible.
- Report research results in a timely manner.
- Report research findings completely and honestly, drawing only those conclusions that are supported by the data presented.
- Report the names of investigators fairly and accurately.
- Interpret the research and the research of others accurately and objectively, drawing conclusions that are supported by the data presented and seeking clarity when uncertain.
- Critically evaluate research methods and results before applying new theory and technology in practice.
- Be knowledgeable concerning currently accepted preventive and therapeutic methods, products, and technology and their application to our practice.

From American Dental Hygienists' Association: *Code of ethics for dental hygienists,* Chicago, 2007-2008, Author.

CHAPTER 6

Ethical Decision Making in Dental Hygiene and Dentistry

PHYLLIS L. BEEMSTERBOER

LEARNING OUTCOMES

- Describe the difference between an issue of right and wrong and a true ethical dilemma.
- Identify the goal for use of an ethical decision-making process in dental hygiene.
- List the six steps provided in the ethical decision-making model.
- List and discuss the categories of common ethical dilemmas for dental hygienists.
- Apply the decision-making model to a hypothetical situation.

KEY TERMS

ethical analysis
ethical dilemma
impaired professional
moral dilemma
moral distress

moral principle
moral sensitivity
moral uncertainty
moral weakness

The student of dental hygiene studies and learns about the ethical and professional responsibilities of a dental hygienist. As a clinician providing care and services, the dental hygienist will be faced with many choices and dilemmas. Some of these choices will be simple issues of right and wrong, whereas others may be *ethical dilemmas* that require careful decision making. The dental hygienist must be aware of the ethical issues that can arise in dental hygiene and dentistry and take appropriate action when necessary. Two aspects are involved in ethics: the ability to discern right from wrong and the commitment to act on a decision.

> *To know what is right and not to do it is the worst cowardice.*
>
> CONFUCIUS

Learning Ethical Decision Making

Ethical problems arise for the dental hygienist in professional practice when the hygienist is caught between two competing obligations. Throughout their lifetimes, professionals face situations that require carefully weighing options. Often no right or wrong answer exists. Instead a variety of answers may be possible, each of which has an element of rightness about it. Most decisions must be made in the context of professional, social, and economic pressures, which may be in conflict with values and principles. Determining what to do when faced with an ethical dilemma can be a daunting challenge. Making such decisions can be greatly facilitated by an ethical decision-making model.

Ethical decision-making models provide a suggested mechanism for critical thinking and resolution of ethical dilemmas. Odom[1] has reported that the usual approach to teaching ethics in dental school and dental hygiene school is either the lecture format or the lecture and case analysis format. He, as well as others, have suggested that students need opportunities to develop the analytical skills needed to assess ethical dilemmas. Odom[2,3] further suggested that posing ethical dilemma cases when a panel of experts is available to help students analyze and arrive at possible solutions to the hypothetical dilemmas is a means of affording those opportunities. The teaching of ethics in dental and dental hygiene educational programs has been acknowledged as an essential part of the education of the dental health care professional. In 1989 the American Dental Education Association (ADEA) established guidelines for all dental-related educational programs that stated curriculum should provide opportunities for refining skills of *ethical analysis* so students are able to apply ethical principles to new and emerging problems in the profession. The goal for these curricula was to develop a commitment by the students to the *moral principles* that are the basis of the profession's contract with society. Moreover, students should be encouraged to develop an attitude that ethical decision making is a process involving lifelong learning and commitment.[4] The ADEA policy has been revised since that time to include expanded statements on professional behavior, societal obligations, access to care needs, and community service.[5]

Intellectual and clinical skills are essential to the competent provision of oral health care, which is why ethics and professionalism are required in the dental hygiene educational curriculum. Effectively fostering and evaluating the ability of students in ethical reasoning and critical thinking is challenging. When faculty are trained in ethical reasoning skills and the authentic evaluation of students, the outcomes are positive; faculty are more comfortable evaluating professional judgment and students report being competent in the skill.[6,7]

▨ Ethical Awareness

How the dental hygienist responds to ethical issues that arise in practice depends on the ethical awareness of the individual *(moral sensitivity)*. A situation or problem can be perceived by one individual as having an ethical component but not by another. In 1993 Campbell and Rogers[8] categorized the kind of moral problems encountered in life and dental practice (Table 6-1). Their first category deals with problems of *moral weakness,* in which moral responsibilities point in one direction and personal inclinations in another. The dental hygienist who forgoes providing a patient with needed dental health education because he or she wants to get to lunch early is lacking in professional responsibility. Another category is *moral uncertainty,* which is defined as the question of whether a moral obligation exists and its scope. For a dental hygienist, dealing with a noncompliant periodontal patient could raise issues of uncertainty. How far should the dental hygienist go to attain a level of health when the patient is unwilling or uninterested in following good dental health advice and guidance? The third category is composed of problems that are *moral dilemmas.* A moral dilemma exists when obligations or responsibilities are in conflict. A large portion of the bioethics literature deals with moral dilemmas that often involve matters of life and death.

TABLE 6-1

Categories of Moral Problems

CATEGORY	CHARACTERISTIC
Moral weakness	Moral responsibilities conflict with personal inclinations
Moral uncertainty	Question as to whether a moral obligation exists
Moral dilemma	Obligations and responsibilities are in conflict
Moral distress	Frustration from perceived powerlessness when what is happening appears to be wrong and are unable to act ethically

Data from Campbell CS, Rogers VC: The normative principles of dental ethics. In Weinstein BD, ed: *Dental ethics*, Philadelphia, 1993, Lea & Febiger.

In order to succeed, you must know what you are doing, like what you are doing, and believe in what you are doing.

WILL ROGERS

The term ***moral distress*** has been added to this listing to acknowledge situations in which the health care provider is frustrated from feelings of powerlessness when a perceived wrong is occurring but he or she is unable to act. It is the feeling experienced when an individual cannot do what he or she believes ought to be done because of a system issue, resistance of a powerful person, or a restraint in the situation. The use of this term came from the nursing profession to describe situations in which the nurse feels powerless to act ethically.[9,10] Although this is a newer term, the resulting distress, emotional toll, anger, guilt, and depression are familiar to many health care providers who must balance conflicts of conscience with professional expectations. An example of this for the dental hygienist could be when treatment recommended by another provider for a patient is deemed excessive or unnecessary. The American Association of Critical Care Nurses (AACCN) advocates a model for rising above moral distress called the "four A's".[11] The goal in this model is to preserve the integrity and authenticity of the health care provider. Addressing moral distress requires making changes (Table 6-2).

▪ Ethical Decision-Making Models

An ethical decision-making model is a tool that can be used by the dental hygienist or other health care provider to help develop the ability to think through an ethical dilemma and arrive at an ethical decision. A number of models are

TABLE 6-2

The "Four A's" to Rise above Moral Distress

TERM	DESCRIPTION
Ask	Ask about distress. Are you showing signs of work-related distress? Become aware of the problem.
Affirm	Affirm your distress and the commitment to take care of yourself. Affirm the professional obligation to act.
Assess	Identify sources of distress and determine severity. Analyze risks and benefits.
Act	Prepare personally and professionally to take action.

Data from American Association of Critical Care Nurses: *AACN public policy position statement: moral distress*, Aliso Viejo, CA, 2008, Author. Available at: www.aacn.org/WD/Practice/Docs/moral_distress.pdf. Accessed September 5, 2008..

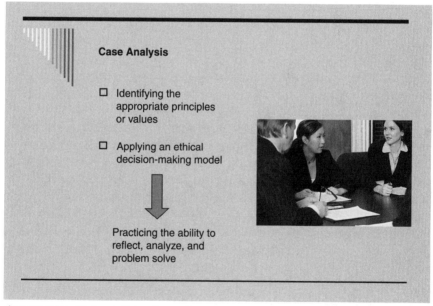

Case Analysis

☐ Identifying the appropriate principles or values

☐ Applying an ethical decision-making model

Practicing the ability to reflect, analyze, and problem solve

Photo copyright Jupiter Images Corporation, 2008.

presented in the ethics literature, all of which are somewhat similar in design and content. The goal of each model is to provide a framework for making the best decision in a particular situation with which the health care provider is confronted. Most of these models use principle-based reasoning, an approach derived from the work of philosophers Beauchamp and Childress.

The model provided in this chapter is a simple six-step approach derived from the decision-making literature as interpreted by Atchison and Beemsterboer and used in the early 1990s with dental and dental hygiene students in a combined

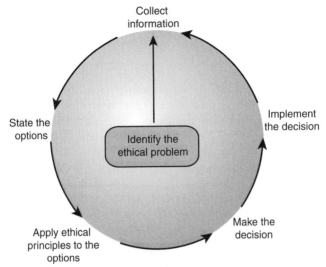

FIGURE 6-1   **Ethical decision-making model.**

ethics course. It is a reasoned approach based on theory and principle. The model has been diagrammed as a circle to emphasize the use of past information and experiences on current and future decision making (Figure 6-1).

The process of decision making is dynamic, evolving as additional information comes into play. Dental hygienists are confronted with myriad questions to consider, requiring them to factor in the code of ethics and their own values and beliefs before arriving at a decision. The evaluation process involved in an ethical dilemma is not unlike that which occurs when the practitioner is faced with a clinical or scientific problem. Careful attention to and systematic analysis of the evidence, facts, and details will help the health care provider reach an appropriate decision. Applying the decision-making model gives the dental hygienist a tool to use throughout professional life.

Six-Step Decision-Making Model

1   Identify the Ethical Dilemma or Problem.   Step 1 is the most critical step in the process. Many situations are simply never perceived to be ethical problems or dilemmas. Once the problem has been recognized, the decision maker must clearly and succinctly state the ethical question, considering all pertinent aspects of the problem. If the ethical question does not place principles in conflict, it is a simple matter of right and wrong and no process of ethical decision making is required. Proceeding to step 2 is not necessary if a clear determination of right or wrong has been made.

2   Collect Information.   The decision maker must gather information to make an informed decision. This may be factual information about the situation as it developed, and it may come from more than one source. Information regarding the values of the parties involved, including those of the health care provider, is needed.

3   State the Options.   After gathering all the necessary information, one may proceed to the third step, which involves brainstorming to identify as many alternatives or options as possible. Often the best decision is not the first one that comes to mind. Also, a tendency exists to think that a question has only one answer. This step forces us to stop and view the situation from all angles to identify what other people might see as alternative answers to the problem. An enlightened and open mind is required to recognize often more than one answer to a problem exists.

4   Apply the Ethical Principles to the Options.   Focus on the ethical principles (autonomy, beneficence, nonmaleficence, and justice) and ethical values and concepts (paternalism, confidentiality, and informed consent). In general, one or more of these will be involved in any ethical decision. State how each alternative will affect the ethical principle or rule by developing a list of pros and cons. In the pro column, show alternatives that protect or hold inviolate each principle or value. In the con column, state how an alternative could violate the principle or value. Do this for each option. This process will enable you to see which ethical principles are in conflict in this situation. Refer to the *ADHA Code of Ethics for Dental Hygienists* for guidance.

5   Make the Decision.   When each alternative has been clearly outlined in terms of pros and cons, a reasonable framework is apparent for making a decision. Each option must then be considered in turn, with attention to how many pros and cons would attend each decision. The seriousness of the cons must then be weighed by the dental hygienist, remembering that, as a professional, he or she is obliged to put the patient's interests first. Simply by examining the options in a careful way, the best solution to an ethical dilemma frequently becomes obvious. Before implementing the decision, the practitioner should replay each principle against the decision to see if the decision holds up to this evaluation.

6   Implement the Decision.   The final step involves acting on the decision that has been made. The decision process will have been futile if no action is taken. Many appropriate decisions are never implemented because this step is omitted. Remember that no action represents tacit approval of a situation.

*T*he man who acts charitably out of a sense of duty is not to be undervalued, but it is the other who most show virtue and therefore to the other that most worth is attributed.

PHILIPPA FOOT

Ethical Dilemmas for the Dental Hygienist

The dental hygienist may be faced with a wide variety of ethical issues and moral dilemmas. A few studies have addressed the responsibility of dental hygienists to report unethical practices. In 1990, Gaston and colleagues conducted a survey of ethical issues in dental hygiene. They found that the three most frequently encountered practice dilemmas were observation of behavior in conflict with standard infection control procedures, failure to refer patients to a specialist, and nondiagnosis of dental disease. One of the conclusions drawn from this study was that serious ethical dilemmas are encountered by most dental hygienists, prompting the authors to advocate increased education of hygienists in the recognition and resolution of ethical problems.

Dentistry, unlike medicine, usually is performed in solo or small group practices where little, if any, institutional oversight is provided by groups such as ethics committees or standard review boards. Dental hygienists usually are employed by a dentist. This arrangement can place the hygienist in a difficult situation when inappropriate care or unethical practices are observed, especially when the dentist employer is involved in the action. In these situations, if the dental hygienist advocates the good of the patient, his or her continued employment may be in jeopardy—thus causing moral distress. Conversely, if the hygienist remains silent, professionalism is compromised and no one speaks for the interests of the patient. This dilemma is similar to what many registered nurses are subjected to when they become advocates for a hospitalized patient.[13] A conflict or dilemma can be intensified when a subordinate observes an unethical action performed by an individual in a position of power. Studies from the nursing literature have reported such situations having a negative impact on the health care environment and leading to burnout and departure from the profession.[11,14] Any type of an ethical dilemma or problem can arise in the practice of dental hygiene. Box 6-1 lists the categories of ethical dilemmas most frequently encountered by dental hygienists.

BOX 6-1

Categories of Ethical Dilemmas Most Commonly Encountered by Dental Hygienists

1 Substandard Care
Situations in which there is failure to diagnose, failure to refer, or lack of proper infection control or in which dental or dental hygiene services are provided that do not meet the accepted standard of care.

2 Overtreatment
Situations in which excessive services or services that are unnecessary for a particular case are provided. This category includes unduly influencing a patient's care decision as a result of one's position of greater knowledge.

3 Scope of Practice
Instances in which the legally assigned scope of practice is exceeded by a dental hygienist, dentist, or other member of the dental team.

4 Fraud
Situations in which an insurance claim or other reimbursement mechanism is adjusted to favor the dental office or the patient's financial situation. Other types of cost-containment efforts may be included in this category.

5 Confidentiality
Situations in which patient and/or child-parent confidentiality is jeopardized or the need and requirement for informed consent is not met.

6 Impaired Professional
Situations in which the dental hygienist or other dental team member cannot or should not perform appropriate dental care because of a dependence on alcohol, drugs, or other substances *(impaired professional)*.

7 Sexual Harassment
Includes a wide range of behaviors that a dental team member may observe or be subjected to that can be classified as harassment.

8 Abuse
Situations in which abuse of a child, elder, or spouse is observed or suspected. Such situations have legal requirements as well as ethical considerations in most states.

> *In any moment of decision, the best thing you can do
> is the right thing. The worst thing you can do
> is nothing.*
>
>   THEODORE ROOSEVELT

Additional types of dilemmas and problems can and will arise. Major advances in technology and the changes in delivery systems in dentistry will further alter the scope and depth of ethical challenges facing dental hygienists and dentists. Dental hygienist also are increasingly finding employment in areas besides private practice, such as research, public health, and corporate fields. These arenas will pose different ethical dilemmas for these individuals.

> *We are what we repeatedly do.*
>
>   ARISTOTLE

Solving a Dilemma Using the Ethical Decision-Making Model

The following hypothetical case is an example of a typical ethical dilemma often faced by a dental hygienist in a private practice situation. This case is presented to illustrate how the ethical decision-making model can be applied to an ethical dilemma.

> Joan Lakeside is a dental hygienist who graduated last year from a dental hygiene program near her hometown. Since graduation, she has been working for a dentist, Dr. Tom McVey, who has been practicing for 20 years. The practice is growing, and Dr. McVey is happy to have Joan working 4 days a week in his busy office. He often tells her how pleased he is with her work and comments how lucky they both were to attend State University Dental School, one of the best in the country.
>
> A patient of the practice, Steve Stafford, is scheduled for an appointment with Joan for the first time. Steve is a 51-year-old white male with normal vital signs, no current medications, and no history of systemic disease. His periodontal condition is good overall, but he does occasionally smoke cigars. Joan notices a small, indurated, white and reddish, slightly raised lesion on the right side of Steve's tongue. On questioning her patient,

Joan finds out that he is unaware of the lesion or how long it has been present in his mouth. Joan shows the lesion to Dr. McVey when he comes into the room to chat with Steve. In earshot of the patient, Dr. McVey tells Joan "not to worry, it is nothing. We'll take a look at it in 6 or 7 months, or whenever Steve gets back in here for his next cleaning."

At the end of the day, Joan goes into Dr. McVey's office and shares with him her concern that the lesion in Steve's mouth looks suspicious and should be referred for biopsy. Once again, Dr. McVey tells her not to worry, adding, "It is my decision as to whether or not we send Steve for a biopsy." Joan is very uncomfortable about the situation and wonders if she should call the patient directly to advise him to seek further examination regarding the lesion on his tongue.

Step 1 in the ethical decision-making model is to identify the dilemma. Joan is concerned about her patient and believes that the lesion on his tongue may be cancerous. Her employer tells her not to be concerned because he does not believe the lesion requires immediate attention. Joan is not reassured because she recalls seeing slides in her pathology class that resemble the lesion on Steve's tongue. Should she call the patient and tell him to seek further examination, or simply forget it and wait until he comes in for his next appointment? That is Joan's ethical dilemma—to call the patient or not.

Steps 2 and 3 involve gathering all pertinent information and listing possible options for action. Joan checks in her oral pathology book and confirms that the lesion on Steve's tongue looks very much like the photographs of squamous cell carcinoma in her text. She identifies the following as her options:

1 Go back to Dr. McVey with her textbook and restate her suspicions in an attempt to convince him to refer the patient for a diagnostic biopsy.
2 Call the patient directly and advise him to seek another opinion about his lesion.
3 Do nothing and wait until the patient comes in for his next appointment.

Step 4 requires that Joan apply the ethical principles and rules to each option she has identified. The first option—talking to Dr. McVey and convincing him to call the patient back in for another examination—applies the principles of nonmaleficence and autonomy. Remove harm is in the patient's best interest, which, in this case, is the possibly cancerous lesion. Option 2—calling the patient directly and advising him to seek care for the lesion—applies the principles of autonomy and beneficence. Autonomy is involved because the patient came in for an examination and has a right to know that he may or may not have a disease. Beneficence—doing good for the patient—is applicable because doing nothing could cause the patient great harm if the lesion were found to be cancerous. The last option—doing nothing and waiting for 6 or 7 months—may involve respecting the autonomy of the dentist.

After completing steps 1 through 4, Joan is prepared for step 5, the decision stage. Joan decides to approach Dr. McVey again and try to convince him to call the patient in for another appointment. If she is unsuccessful in convincing her employer, she will call the patient directly.

Step 6 is implementation. Joan resolves to speak to Dr. McVey first thing the next morning.

The process of ethical decision making can be facilitated by using the decision-making model just described. Numerous other models can be applied to problem solving. Many health care workers find that talking to trusted colleagues and peers about ethical dilemmas and work problems can be both beneficial and comforting. The ethical decision-making model can be applied in a small group and is equally effective for students and experienced practitioners. A sample of a worksheet for assisting in the decision-making process is provided.

> *Let your thoughts be positive for they will become your words. Let your words be positive for they will become your actions. Let your actions be positive for they will become your values. Let your values be positive for they will become your destiny.*
>
> MAHATMA GANDHI

Worksheet for Ethical Decision Making

Step 1

Identify the ethical dilemma. It often helps to phrase the issue in the form of a question. Determine whether it is a right or wrong situation. If so, do not proceed to Step 2.

Steps 2 and 3

List all of the information pertinent to the issue. If legal questions exist, consult an appropriate source for answers. Then state the possible action options that exist. There may be only two, or there may be a long list of options.

Step 4

Apply the ethical principles to each of the options identified. Refer to a listing of ethical principles and rules.

Step 5

State your decision.

Step 6

Implement your decision by taking the appropriate action.

Summary

Ethical choices and dilemmas are bound to occur during the professional life of any health care professional. Ethical decision making, like other aspects of dental hygiene care, can be learned during the education of the dental hygienist and then applied in the practice of dental hygiene. The use of an ethical decision-making model can help the health care professional think through an ethical dilemma and arrive at a decision. The six-step model presented in this chapter can provide structure and guide the dental hygienist when faced with an ethical dilemma.

REFERENCES

1 Odom JG: The status of dental ethics instruction, *J Dent Educ* 52:306, 1988.
2 Odom JG: Recognizing and resolving ethical dilemmas in dentistry, *Med Law* 4:543, 1985.
3 Odom JG, Beemsterboer PL, Pate TD, et al: Revisiting the status of dental ethics instruction, *J Dent Educ* 64:772, 2000.
4 American Association of Dental Schools: Curriculum guidelines on ethics and professionalism in dentistry, *J Dent Educ* 53:144, 1989.
5 American Dental Education Association: *ADEA policy statements,* Washington, DC, 2008, House of Delegates. Available at: www.adea.org/about_adea/governance/Pages/PolicyStatements.aspx. Accessed September 5, 2008.
6 Christie CR, Bowen DM, Paarmann CS: Curriculum evaluation of ethical reasoning and professional responsibility, *J Dent Educ* 67:55, 2003.
7 Christie CR, Bowen DM, Paarmann CS: Effectiveness of faculty training to enhance clinical evaluation of student competence in ethical reasoning and professionalism, *J Dent Educ* 71:1048, 2007.
8 Campbell CS, Rogers VC: The normative principles of dental ethics. In Weinstein BD, ed: *Dental ethics,* Philadelphia, 1993, Lea & Febiger.
9 Corley MC: Nurse moral distress: a proposed theory and research agenda, *Nurs Ethics* 9:636, 2002.
10 Hamric AB, David WS, Childress MD: Moral distress in health care professionals: what is it and what can we do about it? *Pharos* Winter:17, 2006.
11 American Association of Critical Care Nurses: *AACN public policy position statement: moral distress,* Aliso Viejo, CA, 2008, Author. Available at: www.aacn.org/WD/Practice/Docs/moral_distress.pdf. Accessed September 5, 2008.
12 Gaston MA, Brown DM, Waring MB: Survey of ethical issues in dental hygiene, *J Dent Hyg* 64:216, 1990.
13 Redman B, Fry ST: Nurses' ethical conflicts: what is really known about them? *Nurs Ethics* 7:360, 2000.
14 Kalvemark S, Hoglund AT, Hansson MG, et al: Living with conflicts: ethical dilemmas and moral distress in the health care system, *Soc Sci Med* 58A:1075, 2004.

SECTION II

LAW

CHAPTER 7

Society and the State Dental Practice Act

CHERYL A. CAMERON

LEARNING OUTCOMES

- Relate the role of the state in the governing of health care professions.
- Identify the provisions likely to be included in state statutory law for the practice of dental hygiene.
- List the reasons that a dental hygiene license may be suspended, restricted, or revoked.
- Define and describe direct supervision, indirect supervision, and general supervision.
- Recognize the responsibility of the dental hygienist for understanding and observing the state statutory and regulatory provisions.

KEY TERMS

due process
licensure
regulation

scope of practice
statutory law
supervision

State governments are given authority and responsibility to protect the health, safety, and welfare of the state's citizens. The practice of health professionals, including dental hygienists, is governed under this authority. The structure of each state's government is prescribed in the state constitution. In general, state governments are divided into three branches: (1) legislative, (2) executive, and (3) judiciary. The legislative branch is authorized to enact laws or statutes that prescribe or prohibit activities within the state. The executive branch plays a major role in the implementation and enforcement of the prescriptions and prohibitions enacted into law. The judiciary branch is the final arbiter regarding the rights and responsibilities of individuals subject to the laws of the state.

The practice of dental hygiene is regulated through each of these branches of state government. If left unregulated, the practice of dental hygiene could have the potential to harm patients. Dental hygiene is a highly skilled profession that requires professional education for the achievement and maintenance of competence. Government regulation is intended to minimize the public risk of untoward health care outcomes. The state dental practice act is the government regulation that most specifically controls the practice of dental hygiene.

▪ Statutory Law

The legislative branch of government generally is responsible for the enactment of the state dental practice act. In a limited number of states, the state constitution reserves for the people the right to enact laws independent of the legislature. This is the case in the state of Washington, where the constitution provides that:

> The legislative authority of the state of Washington shall be vested in the legislature, consisting of a senate and house of representatives, which shall be called the legislature of the state of Washington, but the people reserve to themselves the power to propose bills, laws, and to enact or reject the same at the polls, independent of the legislature, and also reserve power, at their own option, to approve or reject at the polls any act, item, section, or part of any bill, act, or law passed by the legislature. WASH. CONST. art. II,§1.

Specifically, in 1994, the people of the state of Washington enacted Initiative Measure No. 607, known as the Washington State Denturist Act, whereby:

> The state of Washington finds that to realize the state's current statutory policy of regulating health professions at the least restrictive level consistent

with the public interest, a program of licensure for denturists should be established. The intent of the legislature is to help assure the public's health, provide a mechanism for consumer protection, and offer cost-effective alternatives for denture care services and products to individual consumers and the state. WASH. REV. CODE §18.30.005 (2008).

The state dental practice act may be a single law or a compilation of laws that regulate the practice of dentistry. In the state of Washington, for example, the state dental practice act is a compilation of laws (ch. 18.29 WASH. REV. CODE Dental Hygienist, ch. 18.30 WASH. REV. CODE Denturists, ch. 18.32 WASH. REV. CODE Dentistry, and ch. 18.260 WASH. REV. CODE Dental Professionals) that regulate the practice of dentistry by dentists, dental hygienists, denturists, and dental assistants. Statutes that regulate the health professions are generally not all encompassing. In other words, dental

---

ISSUES THAT MAY BE REGULATED BY STATE LAWS BUT MAY NOT BE SPECIFICALLY INCORPORATED INTO THE STATE DENTAL PRACTICE ACT

- Abuse reporting requirements (e.g., child, dependent adults, and domestic violence)
- Biomedical wastes and hazards management
- Business operation practices (e.g., rebating, credit agreements, business license, and advertising)
- Consent to treatment and informed consent
- Criminal activity
- Disability accommodation
- Education and training requirements (e.g., human immunodeficiency virus [HIV] and blood-borne pathogens)
- False health care claims
- Liability for volunteer services
- Malpractice or actions resulting from health care injuries
- Mandatory malpractice insurance
- Patient confidentiality and heightened protections (e.g., sexually transmitted diseases, mental health treatment, and substance abuse treatment)
- Public health reporting requirements (e.g., contagious or infectious diseases)

hygienists must be familiar with the laws that deal specifically with dental hygiene as well as the general laws that protect the well-being of the state's citizens. For example, most states have enacted laws that require health care professionals to report suspected child abuse. This law may be found in acts that focus on child protection rather than on the practice of dental hygiene. Refer to the box that follows for a list of issues applicable to health care professionals that may be regulated by state law but may not be specifically incorporated into the state dental practice act.

State *statutory law* that regulates the practice of dental hygiene is likely to include provisions regarding the following: (1) licensure requirements, (2) licensure examination requirements, (3) licensure eligibility requirements, (4) licensure by endorsement, (5) approval of educational programs, (6) examination and disciplinary authority, (7) *scope of practice,* (8) supervision requirements, and (9) continuing education requirements. These laws provide a general outline of requirements, provisions, and limitations of the practice of dental hygiene and grant authority to the executive branch of government to implement administrative procedures and requirements. Consider, for example, the following statutory provision, which grants authority to the executive branch of government to establish a continuing education program for dental hygienists:

> In addition to any other authority provided by law, the secretary may:
>
> . . . (7) Establish and implement by rule a continuing education program. WASH. REV. CODE §18.29.130 (2008).

The following rule, implemented by the Washington State Department of Health, establishes the continuing education program applicable to dental hygienists:

> Continuing education for dental hygienists. (1) Purposes. The secretary of the department of health in consultation with the dental hygiene examining committee has determined that the public health, safety and welfare will be served by requiring all holders of dental hygiene licenses granted under chapter 18.29 RCW to continue their education after receiving such licenses. (2) Requirements. Licensed dental hygienists must complete 15 clock hours of continuing education as required in chapter 246-12 WAC, Part 7. A current CPR card must be maintained as part of this requirement. (3) Acceptable continuing education. Continuing education must be dental related education for professional development as a dental hygienist. The 15 clock hours shall be obtained through continuing education courses, correspondence courses, college credit courses, dental hygiene examination standardization/calibration workshops and dental hygiene examination item writer workshops. WASH. ADMIN. CODE §246-815-140 (2008).

▪ Rules and Regulations

The executive branch of government is responsible for implementing the statutory law and providing more specific guidance and *regulation* regarding the practice of dental hygiene. The executive branch includes the departments and agencies of state government (e.g., Department of Health, Department of Professional Regulation, Department of Consumer and Industry Services, or Secretary of State). The development of more specific requirements (e.g., rules) for implementing statutory law is accomplished through a process known as *rule making,* which is a public process that provides the opportunity for input from interested persons, including dental hygienists.

The regulation of the practice of dental hygiene may be facilitated by an appointed board, as in Colorado:

> The state board of dental examiners is hereby created as the agency of this state for the regulation of the practice of dentistry in this state and to carry out the purposes of this article. . . . the board shall consist of seven dentist members, three dental hygienist members, and three members from the public at large, each member to be appointed by the governor for a term of four years . . . COLO. REV. STAT. §12-35-104 (2007).

Alternatively, the practice of dental hygiene may be the purview of an elected regulatory body, as in North Carolina:

> . . . Dental hygienists shall be elected to the Board [of Dental Examiners] in an election . . . in which those persons licensed to practice dental hygiene in North Carolina and residing or practicing in North Carolina shall be entitled to vote. N.C. GEN. STAT. §90-22 (b) (2008).

This body may be referred to in terms such as Board of Dental Examiners, Board of Dentistry, State Dental Board, State Dental Commission, Dental Quality Assurance Commission, or Board of Dental Health Care. Dental hygiene representation on such regulatory bodies is common. The functions of this body may include the examination of dental hygienists for licensure; issuance, renewal, and revocation of dental hygiene licenses; investigation of disciplinary charges; and adoption of rules and regulations regarding the practice of dental hygiene. In some states the regulatory body may be advised by a secondary body, which has greater dental hygiene representation, such as a council, as in Florida, or a Dental Hygienists Committee, as in New Mexico.

> To advise the [Board of Dentistry], it is the intent of the Legislature that councils be appointed as specified in paragraphs (a), (b), and (c) . . . Councils

shall include at least one board member who shall chair the council and shall include nonboard members. All council members shall be appointed by the board chair. Council members shall be appointed for 4-year terms . . . (a) A Council of Dental Hygiene shall be appointed by the board chair and shall include one dental hygienist member of the board, who shall chair the council, one dental member of the board, and three dental hygienists who are actively engaged in the practice of dental hygiene in this state . . . The council is charged with responsibility of and shall meet for the purpose of developing rules and policies for recommendation to the board, which the board shall consider, on matters pertaining to that part of dentistry consisting of educational, preventive, or therapeutic dental hygiene services; dental hygiene licensure, discipline, or regulation; and dental hygiene education. FLA. STAT. ch. §466.004 (2) (2008).

The [New Mexico Board of Dental Health Care] shall ratify the recommendations of the [New Mexico Dental Hygienists Committee] unless the board makes a specific finding that a recommendation is: (1) beyond the jurisdiction of the committee; (2) an undue financial impact upon the board; or (3) not supported by the record. N.M. STAT. ANN. §61-5A-11 (Michie 2008).

The Practice of Dental Hygiene

In the United States the practice of dental hygiene is not nationally regulated and is therefore different in each state. The professional obligation of dental hygienists is to be intimately familiar with the laws and regulations of the state where they practice. A dental hygienist should, on an annual basis, obtain and review the applicable state dental practice act. A good time to do this may be at the time of annual license renewal, birth date, or other annually recurring date of significance. The contact information for the state licensing can be obtained from the American Association of Dental Examiners at www.aadexam.org.

The only good is knowledge and the only evil is ignorance.

SOCRATES

Licensure Provisions

To practice dental hygiene legally, individuals must have a dental hygiene license in the state in which they practice. In general, a condition of dental hygiene *licensure* is graduation from a dental hygiene program accredited by the American Dental Association (ADA) Commission on Dental

Accreditation (CODA) as well as successful completion of a national, regional, and/or state licensure examination.

An exception to these general conditions exists in Alabama, where the law provides for the following:

> Each applicant for examination and license as a dental hygienist shall be a graduate of a school of dental hygiene which has been approved by the board, or in lieu thereof, shall have served at least one year as a dental assistant and shall have served at least one year as a dental hygienist trainee under a training permit issued by the board to a qualified dentist practicing in this state. ALA. CODE §34-9-26 (2008).

A dental hygiene license also may be issued on the basis of a review of credentials, also known as *licensure by endorsement or reciprocity.* Dental hygienists who have graduated from a CODA-accredited dental hygiene program, who are licensed in good standing in a state with similar or higher requirements for licensure, and who have practiced dental hygiene for a minimum prescribed period may have examination requirements waived on the basis of their credentials, as provided for in the following Colorado, North Dakota, and Connecticut statutes:

> The board shall issue a license to an applicant duly licensed as a dental hygienist in another state or territory of the United States who has submitted credentials and qualifications for licensure in Colorado. Such credentials and qualifications shall include: (I) Verification of licensure from any other jurisdiction where the applicant has held a dental hygiene or other health care license; (II) Evidence of the applicant's successful completion of the national board dental examination administered by the joint commission on national dental examinations; (III) Verification that the applicant has been engaged either in clinical practice or in teaching dental hygiene or dentistry in an accredited program for at least one year during the three years immediately preceding the application; (IV) A report of any pending or final disciplinary actions against any health care license held by the applicant at any time; and (V) A report of any pending or final malpractice actions against the applicant. COLO. REV. STAT. §12-35-127(3)(b) (2007).

> Any dental hygienist who is a graduate of a school of dental hygiene which is approved or provisionally approved by the commission on dental accreditation of the American Dental Association and which provides a minimum of two academic years of dental hygiene curriculum, who has been licensed and who has been actively practicing dental hygiene for at least three years prior to the application to practice in this state, who is of good moral character and desirous of removing to this state, who deposits with the board of dental examiners a license from the examining board of the state in which the dental hygienist is licensed, certifying to the fact of

being licensed, and who provides reference letters from three dentists attesting to the dental hygienist's clinical competence, good moral character, and professional attainment, may upon the payment of the fee determined by the board, in the discretion of the board, and upon the satisfactory passing of such examinations as the board deems necessary and proper, be granted a license to practice in this state. N.D. CENT. CODE §43-20-07 (2008).

The Department of Public Health may, without examination, issue a license to any dental hygienist who has provided evidence of professional education not less than that required in this state and who is licensed in some other state or territory, if such other state or territory has requirements of admission determined by the department to be similar to or higher than the requirements of this state, upon certification from the board of examiners or like board of the state or territory in which such dental hygienist was a practitioner certifying to his competency and upon payment of a fee of seventy-five dollars to said department. No license shall be issued under this section to any applicant against whom professional disciplinary action is pending or who is the subject of an unresolved complaint. CONN. GEN. STAT. ANN. §20-126k (LexisNexis 2008).

Some states provide for temporary licensure of dental hygienists who are licensed in other jurisdictions, are relocating to that state, and do not have the option of licensure by credential available to them. A temporary license is valid for a prescribed period or until the next scheduled licensure examination.

Temporary license. (a) The board may issue without examination a temporary license to an applicant for examination who is licensed to practice dental hygiene in another state and who meets the criteria of AS 08.32.030 but who has been in active clinical practice for less than two years immediately preceding application. A temporary license expires at the time notice is given of the results of the next scheduled examination and may not be reissued. ALASKA STAT. §08.32.035 (2008).

A volunteer license may be available to dental hygienists who hold a dental hygiene license in good standing in another jurisdiction, have the minimum specified years of clinical experience, and seek to provide volunteer services.

Restricted volunteer license for certain dentists and dental hygienists. (A) The State Board of Dentistry may issue a restricted volunteer license to a dentist or dental hygienist who: (1) has held the corresponding license in another state as a licensee in good standing; (2) has passed an examination as prescribed by the board; (3) has not failed the state's corresponding clinical examination within the past five years; (4) must have at least five years of clinical practice in the field for which they are seeking the license. (B) A person holding a restricted volunteer license under this section: (1) must only practice in clinics prescribed by the board in regulation; (2) only treat patients who have no insurance or who are not eligible for financial assistance for dental treatment; (3) may not receive remuneration directly or indirectly for providing dental or dental hygiene services. S.C. CODE ANN. §40-15-177 (LexisNexis 2007).

A limited number of states, including Ohio and Maryland, provide for a faculty license for dental hygienists whose practice of dental hygiene is limited to dental hygiene education.

. . . upon application endorsed by an accredited dental hygiene school in this state, the state dental board may without examination issue a teacher's certification to a dental hygienist, authorized to practice in another state or country. A teacher's certificate shall be subject to annual renewal in accordance with the standard renewal procedure . . . and shall not be construed as authorizing anything other than teaching or demonstrating the skills of a dental hygienist in the educational programs of the accredited dental hygiene school which endorsed the application. OHIO REV. CODE ANN. §4715.27 (page 2008).

While it is effective, a teacher's license to practice dental hygiene issued under this title authorizes the licensee to: (1) teach dental hygiene only at the institution named on the license; and (2) practice dental hygiene under the general supervision of a licensed dentist with the institution named on the license. MD. HEALTH OCC. CODE ANN. §4-308(g) (2008).

These licensure provisions are summarized in Table 7-1.

Dental hygienists generally are required to display a current copy of their license at their place(s) of practice.

Every practitioner of . . . dental hygiene . . . shall post and keep conspicuously displayed her or his license in the office wherein she or he practices, in plain sight of the practitioner's patients. Any . . . dental hygienist who practices at more than one location shall be required to display a copy of her or his license in each office where she or he practices. FLA. STAT. ch. §466.016 (2008).

Dental hygiene licenses expire and require renewal on a schedule (e.g., annually) prescribed by state law. When a dental hygienist experiences a limited lapse of licensure (e.g., failure to renew the license before expiration), state law may provide for reinstatement without examination with proof of continued professional competence and payment of renewal and penalty fees, such as in Alaska.

TABLE 7-1

Types of Dental Hygiene Licenses

TYPE OF LICENSE	PURPOSE
Full license	A full dental hygiene license may be granted on the basis of examination or endorsement of credentials; such a license permits unrestricted practice within the scope of the state dental practice act.
Temporary license	A temporary dental hygiene license, granted on the basis of licensure in another jurisdiction, permits practice within the scope of the state dental practice act for a limited period of time while the dental hygienist pursues full licensure status.
Volunteer license	A volunteer dental hygiene license, granted on the basis of licensure in another jurisdiction, permits practice within the scope of the state dental practice act for the purpose of volunteer (e.g., unremunerated) public service.
Faculty license	A faculty dental hygiene license, granted on the basis of prior licensure in another jurisdiction, permits a faculty member to practice within the scope of his or her educational responsibilities.

A licensed dental hygienist who does not pay the renewal registration fee forfeits the hygienist's license. The board may reinstate the license without examination within two years of the date on which payment was due upon written application, proof of continued professional competence, and payment of all unpaid renewal fees and any penalty fee. . . . ALASKA STAT. §08.32.081 (2008).

The practice of dental hygiene without a valid license is a criminal offense.

(1) Each of the following acts constitutes a felony of the third degree . . . (a) Practicing . . . dental hygiene unless the person has an appropriate, active license . . . (b) Using or attempting to use a license . . . which license has been suspended or revoked . . . (2) Each of the following acts constitutes a misdemeanor of the first degree . . . (b) Using the name "dental hygienist" or the initials "R.D.H." or otherwise holding herself or himself out as an actively licensed dental hygienist or implying to any patient or consumer that she or he is an actively licensed dental hygienist unless that person has an active dental hygienist's license. . . . FLA. STAT. ch. §466.026 (2008).

The penalty for noncompliance with licensure requirements may include a monetary fine and/or imprisonment.

> Any person who violates any provision . . . shall be fined not more that five hundred dollars or imprisoned not more than five years or both. Any person who continues to practice dental hygiene or engage as a dental hygienist, after his license or authority to do so has been suspended or revoked and while such disability continues, shall be fined not more than five hundred dollars or imprisoned not more than five years or both. For purposes of this section each instance of patient contact or consultation which is in violation of any provision of this section shall constitute a separate offense. Failure to renew a license in a timely manner shall not constitute a violation for the purposes of this section. CONN. GEN. STAT. ANN. §20-126t (LexisNexis 2008).

A dental hygiene license may be suspended or revoked on the basis of unprofessional conduct, violations of the laws and regulations governing the practice of dental hygiene, and clinical incompetence or the delivery of substandard care. Unprofessional conduct is a broad term that may encompass, but is not limited to, acts of fraud, misrepresentation, or deception; conviction of a felony; aiding and abetting, in the practice of dentistry or dental hygiene, any person not licensed to practice dentistry or dental hygiene; sexual conduct with a patient; and violation of state or federal laws. Dental hygienists also may have their practice restricted or suspended if they become impaired by reason of mental illness, physical illness, or habitual or excessive use or abuse of alcohol or controlled substances.

Many states, such as Florida, have continuing education requirements for maintaining a dental hygiene license.

> In addition to the other requirements for relicensure . . . the board shall require each licensed dental hygienist to complete not less than 24 hours or more than 36 hours of continuing professional education in dental subjects, biennially, in programs prescribed or approved by the board or in equivalent programs of continuing education. FLA. STAT. ch. §466.014 (2008).

Documentation or certification of compliance with continuing education requirements generally is necessary when renewing the license. Renewal of the license also requires payment of a licensing fee. Dental hygienists who are not actively practicing dental hygiene and do not want to maintain a current license may be able to apply for an inactive license. Although not all states have provisions for an inactive status, when available, an inactive license permits a dental hygienist to avoid the expense of maintaining an active license. It also permits the dental hygienist to maintain recognized professional status as a dental hygienist and to reactivate the license upon demonstration of professional competence (e.g., documentation of continuing education). Some states, such as Arkansas, require that a dental hygienist be practicing to maintain active licensure status.

> All licenses issued to dentists and dental hygienists are automatically forfeited if the licensee ceases to practice his profession either in the State of Arkansas or elsewhere for a period of two (2) years. ARK. CODE ANN. §17-82-314 (a)(2008).

Scope of Practice

The scope of dental hygiene practice varies among the states. The practice of dental hygiene includes educational, assessment, preventive, clinical, and other therapeutic services. The specific functions that can be legally performed in each of these aspects of dental hygiene practice are defined by state law. Examples of functions that are routinely allowed to be performed by the dental hygienist include the removal of deposits, accretions, and stains from the supragingival and subgingival surfaces of teeth by scaling, root planing, and polishing; the application of pit and fissure sealants, fluoride, and other topical therapeutic and preventive solutions; dental hygiene examinations and the charting of oral conditions; and exposing, developing, and referring to oral radiographs. The less traditional practice of dental hygiene includes administration of local anesthesia and performance of restorative procedures. This expanded scope of practice may require approved instruction, as in the state of Oregon.

> Expanded Functions of Dental Hygienists. (1) Upon completion of a course of instruction in a program accredited by the Commission on Dental Accreditation of the American Dental Association or other course of instruction approved by the Board, a dental hygienist who completes a Board approved application shall be issued endorsement to perform the following functions under the general supervision of a licensed dentist (a) Administer local anesthetic agents; (b) Use high-speed handpieces to polish restorations; and (c) Apply temporary soft relines to full dentures, providing the patient is seen by the dentist within 14 days after the application. (2) Upon completion of a course of instruction in a program accredited by the Commission on Dental Accreditation of the American Dental Association or other course of instruction approved by the Board, a dental hygienist may administer nitrous oxide under the indirect supervision of a licensed dentist in accordance with the Board's rules regarding anesthesia. OR ADMIN. R. §818-035-0040 (2008).

Restorative Functions of Dental Hygienists. (1) The Board shall issue a Restorative Functions Endorsement (RFE) to a dental hygienist who holds an unrestricted Oregon license, and has successfully completed: (a) A Board approved curriculum from a program accredited by the Commission on Dental Accreditation of the American Dental Association or other course of instruction approved by the Board, and successfully passed the Western Regional Examining Board's Restorative Examination or other equivalent examinations approved by the Board within the last five years; or (b) If successful passage of the Western Regional Examining Board's Restorative Examination or other equivalent examination approved by the Board occurred over five years from the date of application, the applicant must submit verification from another state or jurisdiction where the applicant is legally authorized to perform restorative functions and certification from the supervising dentist of successful completion of at least 25 restorative procedures within the immediate five years from the date of application . . . OR. ADMIN. R. §818-035-0072 (2008).

It may also require a certification separate from the dental hygiene license, as specified in Arkansas statutes.

A dental hygienist shall apply to the board for a certificate to administer local anesthetics. The board shall not issue a certificate until the applicant has met the requirements set forth by the board. ARK. CODE ANN. §17-82-103(c)(2) (2008).

Dental hygienists also are permitted to perform, if competent, any procedure that can legally be delegated to a nonlicensed provider, such as a dental assistant.

A dentist may allow an unlicensed person to perform the following acts under the dentist's close supervision: (1) Oral inspection, with no diagnosis. (2) Patient education in oral hygiene. (3) Place and remove the rubber dam. (4) Hold in place and remove impression materials after the dentist has placed them. (5) Take impressions solely for diagnostic and opposing models. (6) Take impressions and wax bites solely for study casts. (7) Remove the excess cement after the dentist has placed a permanent or temporary inlay, crown, bridge or appliance, or around orthodontic bands. (8) Perform coronal polish. (9) Give fluoride treatments. (10) Place periodontal packs. (11) Remove periodontal packs or sutures. (12) Placement of a matrix and wedge for a silver restoration after the dentist has prepared the cavity. (13) Place a temporary filling (as ZOE) after diagnosis and examination by the dentist. (14) Apply tooth separators as for placement for Class III gold foil. (15) Fabricate, place, and remove temporary crowns or temporary bridges.

(16) Pack and medicate extraction areas. (17) Deliver a sedative drug capsule to patient. (18) Place topical anesthetics. (19) Placement of retraction cord. (20) Polish restorations at a subsequent appointment. (21) Select denture shade and mold. (22) Acid etch. (23) Apply sealants. (24) Place dental x-ray film and expose and develop the films. (25) Take intra-oral and extra-oral photographs. (26) Take health histories. (27) Take and record blood pressure and vital signs. (28) Give preoperative and postoperative instructions. (29) Assist in the administration of nitrous oxide analgesia or sedation . . . (30) Select orthodontic bands for size. (31) Place and remove orthodontic separators. (32) Prepare teeth for the bonding of orthodontic appliances. (33) Fit and adjust headgear. (34) Remove fixed orthodontic appliances. (35) Remove and replace archwires and orthodontic wires. (36) Take a facebow transfer for mounting study casts. WASH. ADMIN. CODE §246-817-520 (2008).

The following functions may be performed by a registered dental hygienist in addition to those authorized pursuant to Sections 1760.5, 1761, 1762, 1763, and 1764: (a) All functions that may be performed by a dental assistant or a registered dental assistant. (b) All persons holding a license as a registered dental hygienist on January 1, 2003, or issued a license on or before December 31, 2005, are authorized to perform the duties of a registered dental assistant specified in Section 1754. All persons issued a license as a registered dental hygienist on and after January 1, 2006, shall qualify for and receive a registered dental assistant license prior to performance of the duties specified in Section 1754. CAL. BUS. & PROF. CODE §1760 (Deering 2007).

General preclusions of practice include diagnosis for dental procedures or treatments, the cutting or removal of hard or soft tissues, and the prescribing of drugs or medications.

Dental hygienists have a legal and professional obligation to limit their practice to the scope of functions permitted by law in the jurisdiction in which they are practicing. If asked by an employing dentist to perform services that are clearly outside the legal scope of practice, the dental hygienist is obligated to decline to comply with the request. If whether a procedure is within the legal scope of practice is unclear, the dental hygienist or employing dentist should seek clarification from the governing authority (e.g., board of dentistry or state dental board).

Supervision Requirements

The level of *supervision* required for the practice of dental hygiene varies by state, scope of practice, and location of practice. Although the specific definitions for supervision are state specific, they can be generalized. Direct supervision generally requires prior diagnosis of the patient's condition and authorization of a procedure by a dentist, the presence of a supervising dentist on the premises, and dentist approval of the work performed before patient dismissal. Indirect supervision requires prior diagnosis of the patient's condition and authorization of a procedure by a dentist and the presence of a supervising dentist on the premises. General supervision requires that the services being delivered be authorized by the dentist; however, the presence of the supervising dentist in the treatment facility is not required. Some states, such as Alaska, require dental hygienists to report the name and address of the dentist under whose supervision they are practicing.

> Every dental hygienist practicing dental hygiene in the state shall furnish the board with the name and address of the dentist under whose supervision the dental hygienist is practicing. ALASKA STAT. §08.32.130 (2008).

A limited number of states, including Colorado, Connecticut, New Mexico, and Minnesota, permit some form of unsupervised practice of dental hygiene.

> What constitutes practicing unsupervised dental hygiene. (1) Unless licensed to practice dentistry, any person shall be deemed to be practicing unsupervised dental hygiene who: (a) Removes deposits, accretions, and stains by scaling with hand, ultrasonic, or other devices from all surfaces of the tooth and smooths and polishes natural and restored tooth surfaces; (b) Removes granulation and degenerated tissue from the gingival wall of the periodontal pocket through the process of gingival curettage; (c) Provides preventive measures including the application of fluorides, sealants, and other recognized topical agents for the prevention of oral disease; (d) Gathers and assembles information including, but not limited to, fact-finding and patient history, oral inspection, and dental and periodontal charting; or (e) Administers a topical anesthetic to a patient in the course of providing dental care. (2) Unsupervised dental hygiene may be performed by licensed dentists and licensed dental hygienists without the supervision of a licensed dentist. COLO. REV. STAT. §12-35-124 (2007).
>
> No person shall engage in the practice of dental hygiene unless such person (1) has a dental hygiene license issued by the Department of Public Health and (A) is practicing under the general supervision of a licensed dentist, or (B) has been practicing as a licensed dental hygienist for at least two years, is practicing in a public health facility and complies with the requirements of subsection (e) of this section . . . (f) Each dental hygienist practicing in a public health facility shall (1) refer for treatment any patient

with needs outside the dental hygienist's scope of practice, and (2) coordinate such referral for treatment to dentists. . . . CONN. GEN. STAT. ANN. §20-126l(b) (LexisNexis 2008).

For the purpose of this section, "collaborative practice of dental hygiene" means the application of the science of prevention and treatment of oral disease through the provision of educational, assessment, preventive, clinical and other therapeutic services . . . in a cooperative working relationship with a consulting dentist, but without general supervision . . . N.M. STAT. ANN. §61-5A-4(F) (Michie 2008).

Limited authorization for dental hygienists. (a) . . . a dental hygienist licensed under this chapter may be employed or retained by a health care facility, program, or nonprofit organization to perform dental hygiene services described under paragraph (b) without the patient first being examined by a licensed dentist if the dental hygienist: (1) has been engaged in the active practice of clinical dental hygiene for not less than 2,400 hours in the past 18 months or a career total of 3,000 hours, including a minimum of 200 hours of clinical practice in two of the past three years; (2) has entered into a collaborative agreement with a licensed dentist that designates authorization for the services provided by the dental hygienist; (3) has documented participation in courses in infection control and medical emergencies within each continuing education cycle; and (4) maintains current certification in advanced or basic cardiac life support as recognized by the American Heart Association, the American Red Cross, or another agency that is equivalent to the American Heart Association or the American Red Cross. MN STAT §150A.10 (LexisNexis 2007).

Other Selected Statutory Provisions

Not all laws governing the practice of dental hygiene are encompassed in the state dental practice act. This does not negate, however, the dental hygienist's obligation to comply with such laws. This section provides examples of laws that may not be incorporated in the state dental practice act but instead may be located in other statutes that are universally applicable to health care providers or by topic (e.g., child protection statutes).

Abuse Reporting

Most states have enacted laws that mandate the reporting of child abuse.

In order to protect children whose health and well-being may be adversely affected through the infliction, by other than accidental means, of harm through physical injury or neglect, mental injury, sexual abuse, sexual exploitation, or maltreatment, the legislature requires the reporting of these cases by practitioners of the healing arts and others to the department. It is not the intent of the legislature that persons required to report suspected child abuse or neglect under the chapter investigate the suspected child abuse or neglect before they make the required report to the department. Reports must be made when there is a reasonable cause to suspect child abuse or neglect in order to make state investigative and social services available in a wider range of cases at an earlier point in time, to make sure that investigations regarding child abuse and neglect are conducted by trained investigators, and to avoid subjecting a child to multiple interviews about the abuse or neglect. ALASKA STAT. §47.17.010 (2008).

In addition, several states, including Colorado, have enacted legislation that mandates or encourages the reporting of abuse of vulnerable, dependent, and disabled adults.

An immediate oral report of abuse should be made or caused to be made within twenty-four hours to the county department or during non-business hours to a local law enforcement agency responsible for investigating violations of state criminal laws protecting at-risk adults by any person specified in paragraph (b) of this subsection (1) who has observed the mistreatment or self-neglect of an at-risk adult or who has reasonable cause to believe that an at-risk adult has been mistreated or is self-neglected and is at imminent risk of mistreatment or self-neglect. (b) The following persons are urged to make or initiate an initial oral report within twenty-four hours followed by a written report within forty-eight hours: (I) Physicians, surgeons, physicians' assistants, or osteopaths, including physicians in training; (II) Medical examiners or coroners; (III) Registered nurses or licensed practical nurses; (IV) Hospital and nursing home personnel engaged in the admission, care, or treatment of patients; (V) Psychologists and other mental health professionals; (VI) Social work practitioners; (VII) Dentists; (VIII) Law enforcement officials and personnel; (IX) Court-appointed guardians and conservators; (X) Fire protection personnel; (XI) Pharmacists; (XII) Community-centered board staff; (XIII) Personnel of banks, savings and loan associations, credit unions, and other lending or financial institutions; (XIV) State and local long-term care ombudsmen; (XV) Any caretaker, staff member, or employee of or volunteer or consultant for any licensed care facility, agency, home, or governing board. COLO. REV. STAT. §26-3.1-102 (1)(a) (2007).

Dental hygienists should be familiar with their personal responsibility to report abuse.

All that is necessary for evil to triumph is for good people to do nothing.

EDMUND BURKE

Patient Records

Although the maintenance of a patient record is professionally prudent, it may also be mandated statutorily. Some states have incorporated patient record requirements within the state dental practice act or related regulations (e.g., WASH. ADMIN. CODE §246-817-310 [2008]), whereas others have enacted separate laws that broadly delineate the requirements for maintaining health care information (e.g., ch. 50-16 MONT. CODE ANN. Uniform Health Care Information and NEV. REV. STAT. ANN. §629.051 [2008]). Health care records are generally recognized to be confidential and protected against disclosure to unauthorized third parties (e.g., ch. 5-37.3 R.I. GEN. LAWS Confidentiality of Health Care Communications and Information Act).

Professional Liability Insurance

Dental hygienists in some states are mandated to maintain professional liability insurance or other indemnity against liability for professional malpractice. When mandated, the law may prescribe the level of insurance that must be maintained per incident as well as in the aggregate.

> Each person licensed to practice dental hygiene under the provisions of this chapter who provides direct patient care services shall maintain professional liability insurance or other indemnity against liability for professional malpractice. The amount of insurance that each such person shall carry as insurance or indemnity against claims for injury or death for professional malpractice shall not be less than five hundred thousand dollars for one person, per occurrence, with an aggregate of not less than one million five hundred thousand dollars. CONN. GEN. STAT. ANN. §20-126x (a) (LexisNexis 2008).

Cardiopulmonary Resuscitation Certification

Maintaining current cardiopulmonary resuscitation (CPR) certification is professionally prudent. In addition, some states have enacted legislation that mandates that dental professionals be currently certified in CPR.

Self-Referral and Kickbacks

State and local self-referral statutes have been enacted to avoid the conflict of interest that may be inherent in the referral of a patient by a health care provider to a provider of health care services in which the referring provider has an investment interest (e.g., FLA. STAT. ch. §456.053 [2008]). Prohibitions on kickbacks, or remuneration or payment back as an incentive or inducement to refer or solicit patients, also have been enacted at the federal and state levels (e.g., FLA. STAT. ch. §456.054 [2008]).

Due Process

In the event of threatened adverse actions against licensure status, dental hygienists should become familiar with the available administrative procedures. General *due process* provisions include notice and an opportunity to be heard. Notice generally includes a statement of the proposed action to be taken, the available evidence supporting the proposed action, and the opportunity for a hearing. The proposed action can be taken uncontested if the dental hygienist fails to respond within the time and in the manner specified in the notice. If a hearing is requested, the dental hygienist will be notified, at a minimum, of the time and place of the hearing and who will conduct the hearing.

The law is not an end itself, nor does it provide ends. It is preeminently a means to serve what we think is right.

WILLIAM J. BRENNAN, JR.

Summary

Dental hygiene is a state-regulated health profession because of society's concern for the well-being of its citizens. The dental hygiene professional is obligated to be intimately familiar with the statutory and regulatory provisions of the practice of dental hygiene. Noncompliance with these provisions is not an excuse for failure to know or understand one's professional responsibilities. Therefore, on an annual basis, dental hygiene professionals should obtain a current copy of the state dental practice act for the jurisdiction(s) in which they are licensed and practicing.

Honor is like a rugged island without a shore; once you have left it, you cannot return.

NICOLAS BOILEAU

CHAPTER 8

Dental Hygienist–Patient Relationship

CHERYL A. CAMERON
AND PAMELA ZARKOWSKI

LEARNING OUTCOMES

- Describe the professional obligation that exists between the dental hygienist and the patient.
- Recognize the difference between civil law and criminal law in the U.S. legal system.
- Compare intentional torts and persons, intentional torts and property, and unintentional torts of negligence.
- List and evaluate the rights and responsibilities of the dental hygienist in the provider-patient relationship.
- State the patient's responsibilities when receiving oral health care.
- Describe the elements of informed consent.
- Define *malpractice* and *contributory negligence*.

KEY TERMS

abandonment	*criminal law*	*injury*
allegation	*defamation*	*injury causation*
battery	*defendant*	*intentional tort*
breach of contract	*deposition*	*malpractice*
civil action	*discovery*	*negligence*
civil law	*emancipated*	*sanction*
contributory	*minor*	*statute of limitations*
negligence	*fiduciary relationship*	*tort*
criminal action	*informed consent*	*unintentional tort*

The dental hygienist–patient relationship is a critical factor in the delivery of quality dental hygiene care. The dental hygienist–patient relationship is a two-party association that can only achieve its fullest potential with the committed participation of each of the parties. Patients enter the relationship with certain expectations. Dental hygienists must understand these expectations through communication with their patients. If dental hygienists are unable to meet their patients' expressed expectations, the patients must understand this limitation and either accept the limitation and alter their expectations or seek care from an alternative provider who is able to meet the expectations. The dental hygienist has a professional obligation in this relationship to comply with the laws that govern the practice of dental hygiene and to deliver oral health care services that meet the standards of care of the profession. Failure to fulfill this professional obligation can result in untoward consequences to the patient and dental hygienist. The consequences to the patient may be substandard and/or unauthorized care. Several consequences for the dental hygienist are possible, as follows:

- Complaint review, as provided in the Missouri statute that follows:

  The board may cause a complaint to be filed with the administrative hearing commission as provided by chapter 621, RSMo, against any holder of any permit or license required by this chapter . . . for any one or any combination of the following causes: (1) Use of any controlled substance . . . or alcoholic beverage to an extent that such use impairs a person's ability to perform the work of any professional licensed or regulated by this chapter; (2) The person has been finally adjudicated and found guilty . . . in a criminal prosecution . . . (3) Use of fraud, deception, misrepresentation or bribery in securing any permit or license issued pursuant to this chapter . . . (4) Obtaining or attempting to obtain any fee, charge, tuition or other compensation by fraud, deception or misrepresentation . . . (5) Incompetency, misconduct, gross negligence, fraud, misrepresentation or dishonesty in the performance of, or relating to one's ability to perform, the functions or duties of any profession licensed or regulated by this chapter; (6) Violation of, or assisting or enabling any person to violate, any provision of this chapter . . . (7) Impersonation of any person holding a permit or license or allowing any person to use his or her permit, license or diploma from any school; (8) Disciplinary action against the holder of a license or other right to practice any profession regulated by this chapter imposed by another state, province, territory, federal agency or country upon grounds for which discipline is authorized by this state; (9) A person is finally adjudicated incapacitated or disabled by a court of competent jurisdiction; (10) Assisting or enabling any person to practice or offer to practice, by lack of supervision or in any other manner, any profession licensed or regulated by the chapter . . . (11) Issuance of a permit or license based upon a material mistake of fact; (12) Failure to display a valid certificate, permit or license if so required . . . (13) Violation of any professional trust or confidence; (14) Use of any advertisement or solicitation that is false, misleading or deceptive . . . (15) Violation of the drug law . . . (16) Failure or refusal to properly guard against contagious, infectious or communicable diseases or the spread thereof; (17) Failing to maintain his or her office or offices, laboratory, equipment and instruments in a safe and sanitary condition; (18) Accepting, tendering or paying "rebates" to or "splitting fees" with any other person . . . (19) Administering, or causing or permitting to be administered, nitrous oxide gas in may amount to himself or herself, or to another unless as an adjunctive measure to patient management; (20) Being unable to practice as a . . . hygienist with reasonable skill and safety to patients by reasons of professional incompetency, or because of illness, drunkenness, excessive use of drugs, narcotics, chemicals, or as a result of any mental or physical condition. MO. ANN. STAT §332.321 (2) (LexisNexis 2008).

- Disciplinary *sanctions* such as those provided in the following Nevada statute:

  . . . The [Board of Dental Examiners] may: (a) Refuse to issue a license to any person; (b) Revoke or suspend the license or renewal certificate issued by it to any person; (c) Fine a person it has licensed; (d) Place a person on probation for a specified period on any conditions the Board may order; (e) Issue a public reprimand to a person; (f) Limit a person's practice to certain branches of dentistry; (g) Require a person to participate in a program to correct alcohol or drug abuse or any other impairment; (h) Require that a person's practice be supervised; (i) Require a person to perform public service without compensation; (j) Require a person to take a physical or mental examination or an examination of his competence; (k) Require a person to fulfill certain training or educational requirements; or (l) Require a person to reimburse a patient; or (m) Any combination thereof, upon submission of substantial evidence to the Board that the person has engaged in any of the activities listed in subsection 2. 2. The following activities may be punished as provided in subsection 1: (a) Engaging in the illegal practice of dentistry or dental hygiene; (b) Engaging in unprofessional conduct; or (c) Violating any regulations adopted by the Board or the provisions of this chapter. NEV. REV. STAT. §631.350 (2008).

- Criminal penalties (such as provided in the following Nevada statute) and/or civil legal action:

  A person who practices or offers to practice dental hygiene in this State without a license, or who, having a license, practices dental hygiene in a manner or place not permitted by the provisions of this chapter: (a) If it is his first or second offense, is guilty of a gross misdemeanor, (b) If it is his third or subsequent offense, is guilty of a category D felony. NEV. REV. STAT. §631.400 (2) (2008).

- Other possible consequences, including discontinuation of the patient relationship or loss of employment

Legal Framework of the Relationship

In addition to being a professional relationship, the dental hygienist–patient relationship also is legally binding. Dental hygiene professionals must be familiar with the legal principles of the dental hygienist–patient relationship to guide their actions, decisions, record keeping, and professional interactions. The legal principles are based on society's general belief that citizens have a right to be protected and, if they come to harm at the hands of another, they have a right to be compensated.

Society provides for retribution to harmed citizens through civil and criminal litigation (*civil action* or *criminal action*). A civil offense is a wrongful act against a person that violates his or her person (body), privacy, or property or contractual rights. A dental hygienist who fails to provide appropriate periodontal therapy, resulting in a condition of increased severity, may have committed a civil offense. An office manager who breaches confidentiality by discussing a patient's medical condition with an unauthorized person without the patient's consent may have committed a civil offense. A violation of *criminal law* is a violation of a societal rule outlined by statutory law. Physically harming someone with a weapon is a criminal offense, as is practicing dental hygiene without a license. Although civil offenses are most commonly litigated, both civil and criminal offenses can be committed in the practice of dental hygiene.

> *O*ur character is revealed by how we treat people who cannot help us or hurt us.
>
> MICHAEL JOSPEHSON

Overview of the Legal System

The legal system has a clearly outlined structure for dealing with civil and criminal offenses, including filing, investigating, and resolving claims and *allegations.* The party bringing a claim is referred to as the *plaintiff* in a civil proceeding and the *prosecutor* in a criminal proceeding. The party defending a claim is referred to as the **defendant.** The investigation of claims and allegations includes the **discovery** of evidence, which may be gathered through interrogatories and **depositions.** In addition to the plaintiff (i.e., harmed party) and defendant, other individuals who may be witnesses to events or recorders of information may be called on to respond to requests for information. The resolution of claims and allegations may require a court proceeding known as a *trial.* In a trial, the plaintiff or prosecutor is given the opportunity to present allegations, including evidence, and the defendant is given an opportunity to present a defense, including evidence, to a panel of judges or jury. Questions of law are decided by judges, whereas questions of fact are decided by juries. In a criminal case, the establishment of guilt requires a high level of certainty known as *beyond a reasonable doubt.* In a civil case, the establishment of a claim may require a level of certainty that is greater than 50%, known as the *preponderance of evidence.* The nature of the claim or allegation influences the determination of which party (plaintiff or defendant) bears the responsibility for meeting the required level of proof.

Civil Law

The two major categories of *civil law* are contract law and tort law.

Contract Law

A contract is a legally binding agreement to keep a promise in exchange for something of value. The courts view the relationship between a health care provider and a patient in terms of a contract. Simply stated, a dental provider agrees to deliver oral health care services to a patient and, in return, the patient agrees to cooperate in the care and arrange for appropriate payment (a *fiduciary relationship*). The exchange of promises that creates a binding contract may be express or implied. An express contract is an agreement that is stated in explicit language, either orally or in writing. For example, a written treatment plan that outlines the procedures to be performed and associated costs for the delivery of those procedures may be viewed as an express contract. An implied contract is recognized if, based on the circumstances surrounding a particular event, the assumption that a contract exists between the parties is reasonable. In a dental office, the patient's action of arriving at the office at a scheduled time and sitting in the dental chair, and the dental provider's actions of treating the patient, may establish an implied contract. A contractual relationship is a multisided relationship that binds each of the parties to fulfill their committed responsibilities. Failure to meet one's contractual obligations is known as a *breach of contract,* which may be remedied through the judicial system.

Tort Law

A *tort* is a civil wrong that results from breach of a legal duty that exists by virtue of society's expectations of performance, rather than a contractual or privately created performance obligation. Torts include two types: intentional and unintentional. An *intentional tort* is a deliberate and purposeful act that has substantial certainty of untoward consequences from the act. Intentional torts relate to persons and to property. Insurance policies that protect health care providers against liability associated with the delivery of health care may not provide coverage for intentional tort liability. An *unintentional tort* includes no intent to cause harm, although harm or *injury* does occur.

Intentional Torts to Persons. The intentional tort of *battery* is defined as harmful, nonconsensual, or offensive contact with a person. An injury does not have to occur, only a physical invasion of a person. Intentional torts are differentiated from unintentional torts on the basis of the state of mind of the perpetrator and his or her intent to cause harm. For example, a dental hygienist who slaps a child on his buttocks with the intent to make physical contact and punish the child for difficult behavior may be guilty of battery. An assault is an action that causes apprehension in a person. No physical contact occurs in an assault, but the action may involve words and conduct. For example, a dental hygienist who raises his or her voice and threatens to harm a patient with a dental instrument, creating fear and apprehension on the part of the patient that a battery may occur, may be guilty of an assault. Dental hygienists must therefore use caution in patient management techniques to minimize the risk of being accused of battery or assault. Methods of restraint should be selected carefully, and permission should be granted before use.

Misrepresentation is another category of intentional tort. Misrepresentation is an incorrect or false representation. Consider, for example, the situation in which an office dental hygienist calls in sick on a day that is completely scheduled with patients. If the employer dentist allows the dental assistant, who is a dental hygiene student, to be the "dental hygienist for the day," this action is a purposeful misrepresentation because patients believe they are being treated by a dental hygienist who is licensed and qualified.

Other intentional torts include false imprisonment involving restraint against a victim's will, intentional infliction of emotional distress through an act of extreme and outrageous conduct, and slander or *defamation* causing damage to the reputation of another.

Intentional Torts to Property. The physical invasion of intruding on land without authorization is a form of intentional tort. Interference with the possession of an individual's property is another form of intentional tort. For example, finding a colleague's lost handpiece and keeping it as one's own property is interference.

Unintentional Tort of Negligence. *Negligence* is an unintentional tort that involves the failure to act as a reasonable, prudent person under similar circumstances. Malpractice is a form of negligence that, in the context of medicine and dentistry, includes all liability-producing conduct resulting from the delivery of health care services.

▪ Rights and Responsibilities of the Dental Hygienist and Patient

The dental hygienist–patient relationship includes a number of rights and responsibilities for both parties (Boxes 8-1 and 8-2). Failure by either party to meet its obligations can result in litigation. Dental hygienists must become familiar with their responsibilities to patients, which include the following:

- Dental hygienists must have a current license for the state in which they practice and have it displayed as required. An individual who fails to renew a license or who is denied a license cannot practice. Dental hygienists must perform only the legally allowed duties with appropriate supervision.
- Dental hygienists must deliver care that meets the standard of a reasonable person in the profession. A reasonable person is one who would use suitable judgment based on the circumstances. A practitioner makes a judgment or decision based on his or her educational training and experience. A dental hygienist is held to the standard of a dental hygienist, not a dentist or a physician.
- A dental hygienist must use drugs, materials, and techniques recognized by the profession. Patients trust that the dental hygienist will recommend or use therapeutic treatments recognized by professional groups, such as the American Dental Association (ADA) or the American Academy of Periodontology (AAP).
- An office must complete treatment in a timely manner. An office that chooses to delay or extend treatment for any reason, such as in the case of a patient with a difficult personality, is at risk of extending treatment beyond an acceptable time.

> **BOX 8-1**
>
> ## The Dental Hygienist's Responsibilities When Delivering Oral Health Care
>
> - Possess a proper license and registration, comply with all laws, and practice within the scope of practice as dictated by state law.
> - Exercise reasonable skill, care, and judgment in the assessment, diagnosis, and treatment of patients.
> - Use standard drugs, materials, and techniques.
> - Complete treatment within a reasonable time.
> - Charge reasonable fees.
> - Never abandon a patient, and always arrange for care during absence.
> - Refer unusual cases to a specialist.
> - Maintain patient privacy and confidentiality.
> - Keep accurate records.
> - Give adequate instructions to the patient.
> - Maintain a level of knowledge and practice within the code of ethics.

> **BOX 8-2**
>
> ## Patient Responsibilities When Receiving Oral Health Care
>
> - Pay a reasonable fee in a reasonable time.
> - Cooperate in care and keep appointments.
> - Provide accurate answers about dental or medical history and current health status.
> - Follow instructions, including home care instruction.

- An office should charge fees that are usual, customary, and reasonable.
- An office cannot stop treatment of a patient if harm will occur. The discontinuation of the provider-patient relationship requires appropriate notification to avoid **abandonment.** The necessary notification includes informing the patient in writing, allowing emergency care to be provided for a specific period, suggesting that the patient seek another provider, and providing the patient with an opportunity to obtain his or her dental records. An office also must have a policy

for short-term absence. To meet this obligation, a dental office may use an answering service, voice mail, or pagers to allow emergency contact.

- A dental hygienist has a duty to understand his or her abilities and limitations and to refer patients elsewhere when appropriate.
- A dental hygienist must respect a patient's right to privacy. Patient information can be shared with unauthorized parties only with the patient's permission. Office staff must be careful not to divulge information without a patient's consent. Office staff also must be cautious not to have casual or public conversations about a patient that would violate the patient's privacy.
- An office is required to record information received in a manner that is logical, complete, and accurate. Records may include written documentation (e.g., collected data, diagnoses, treatment plans, and a description of the treatment provided), radiographs, and models. Patients have the right to obtain a copy of their records.
- An office must give the patient appropriate and understandable pretreatment and posttreatment instructions. Instructions may be provided verbally and in writing. In offices with diverse patient populations, instructions should be available in frequently spoken languages to facilitate understanding.
- Dental hygienists are required to remain current with all aspects of patient care. Attending continuing education courses, reading scientific literature, and using other educational sources to keep knowledge and skill levels up to date are important. In addition, an awareness of and adherence to a professional code of ethics are imperative.

Patients in a dental office expect to receive quality care. Patients seek care, trusting that their legal rights will not be violated and that their health and oral health status will not be harmed. When harm or injury does occur, a number of remedies may be available through the judicial system.

▪ Legal Actions for Health Care Injuries

When the care delivered by a dental hygienist results in injury, the injured patient may seek compensation and retribution through the courts. The three most common actions relating to health care are (1) failure to obtain informed consent, (2) professional malpractice, and (3) breach of contract. At the core of each of these actions is the question of whether the dental hygienist violated a duty owed to the patient. The American Dental

Hygienists' Association (ADHA) recognizes that the dental hygienist has the following professional responsibilities to patients*:

- Provide oral health care using high levels of professional knowledge, judgment, and skill.
- Maintain a work environment that minimizes the risk of harm.
- Serve all [patients] without discrimination and avoid action toward any individual or group that may be interpreted as discriminatory.
- Hold professional [patient] relationships confidential.
- Communicate with [patients] in a respectful manner.
- Promote ethical behavior and high standards of care by all dental hygienists.
- Serve as an advocate for the welfare of [patients].
- Provide [patients] with the information necessary to make informed decisions about their oral health and encourage their full participation in treatment decisions and goals.
- Refer [patients] to other health care providers when their needs are beyond [the dental hygienist's] ability or scope of practice.
- Educate patients about high-quality oral health care.

To teach is to learn.

JAPANESE PROVERB

Informed Consent

History.   An essential step in understanding and meeting the expectations of a patient involves obtaining the patient's informed consent before the delivery of oral health care services. *Informed consent* is based on the premise that every citizen has the basic right to be free from invasions of their body without permission. This premise was strongly asserted by the United States Supreme Court in 1891 in *Union Pacific Railway v. Botsford,* 141 U.S. 250, 251 (1891), when it stated that "No right is held more sacred, or is more carefully guarded, by the common law, than the right of every individual to the possession and control of his own person, free from all restraint or interference of others, unless by clear and unquestionable authority of law." This position was extended to the delivery of health care in 1914 in

---

* Excerpted from American Dental Hygienists' Association: *Code of ethics for dental hygienists,* Chicago, 2007-2008, Author. The use of the term *client* in the code has been replaced with *patient.*

Schloendorff v. Society of New York Hospital, 105 N.E. 92, 93 (1914), when the court opined that "Every human being of adult years and sound mind has a right to determine what shall be done with his own body; and a surgeon who performs an operation without his patient's consent commits an assault."

Over time, the concept of consent to health care evolved into the concept of informed consent. Informed consent balances the health care provider's unique knowledge and skill with the patient's decision-making role by placing an affirmative duty on the health care provider to disclose the nature of a procedure to be performed as well as the risks and benefits of proposed and alternative treatment. The concept of informed consent was first expressed in 1957 in *Salgo v. Leland Stanford Jr. Univ. Bd. of Trustees,* 317 P.2d 170 (Cal. Ct. App. 1957), when the court held that formal and documented consent was legally ineffective if the patient lacked an understanding of material information about the treatment being authorized. Although informed consent was first addressed in common law (i.e., the reported opinions of courts, also known as *case law*), the doctrine of informed consent also has been codified through state statutory enactments. In addition to a legal obligation to obtain informed consent, the ADHA also recognizes an ethical obligation, as specified in the following excerpt from its *Code of Ethics for Dental Hygienists:*

> Individual autonomy and respect for human beings—People have the right to be treated with respect. They have the right to informed consent prior to treatment, and they have the right to full disclosure of all relevant information so that they can make informed choices about their care.

Elements of Informed Consent. Individuals who incur a health care injury and allege that they were not adequately informed regarding the procedure to which they consented may file a legal action against the dental hygienist for failure to obtain informed consent. To be successful in establishing a cause of action for failure to obtain informed consent, a patient must generally establish (1) that the dental hygienist had a duty to disclose sufficient information about the proposed treatment to obtain the patient's informed consent, (2) that the dental hygienist breached that duty, and (3) that the dental hygienist's breach of duty was the cause of the injury sustained by the patient.

A duty to disclose information arises when a potential danger or risk is associated with a proposed treatment that may influence the decision whether to proceed with the treatment. Two different standards have emerged as the general measure of the duty to disclose: (1) professional community standard and (2) materiality standard. The professional community standard (see the North Carolina and Kentucky statutes that follow) is based on the accepted practice of the professional community, whereas the materiality standard (see the Washington statute that follows) is based on the needs of the patient to make an autonomous and informed treatment decision. The dental hygienist must be familiar with the informed consent statutes in the jurisdiction of practice as well as the judicial interpretations of the statutory language.

Informed consent to health care treatment or procedure. (a) No recovery shall be allowed against any health care provider upon the grounds that the health care treatment was rendered without the informed consent of the patient or other person authorized to give consent for the patient where: (1) The action of the health care provider in obtaining the consent of the patient or other person authorized to give consent for the patient was in accordance with the standards of practice among members of the same health care profession with similar training and experience situated in the same or similar communities. N.C. GEN. STAT. §90-21.13 (2008).

Informed consent—When deemed given. In any action brought for treating, examining, or operating on a claimant wherein the claimant's informed consent is an element, the claimant's informed consent shall be deemed to have been given where: (1) The action of the health care provider in obtaining the consent of the patient or another person authorized to give consent for the patient was in accordance with the accepted standard of medical or dental practice among members of the profession with similar training and experience. KY. REV. STAT. ANN. §304.40-320 (2008).

Failure to secure informed consent—Necessary elements of proof— Emergency situations. (1) The following shall be necessary elements of proof that injury resulted from health care in a civil negligence or arbitration involving the issue of the alleged breach of the duty to secure an informed consent by a patient or his representatives against a health care provider: (a) That the health care provider failed to inform the patient of a material fact or facts relating to the treatment; (b) That the patient consented to the treatment without being aware of or fully informed of such material fact or facts; (c) That a reasonably prudent patient under similar circumstances would not have consented to the treatment if informed of such material fact or facts; (d) That the treatment in question proximately caused injury to the patient. (2) Under the provisions of this section a fact is defined as or considered to be a material fact, if a reasonably prudent person in the position of the patient or his representative would attach significance to it deciding whether or not to submit to the proposed treatment. (3) Material facts under the provisions of this section which must be established by expert testimony shall be either: (a) The nature and character of the treatment proposed and administered; (b) The anticipated results of the treatment proposed and administered; (c) The recognized possible alternative forms of treatment; or (d) The recognized serious possible risks, complications, and anticipated benefits involved in the treatment administered and in the recognized possible alternative forms of treatment, including nontreatment. (4) If a recognized health care emergency exists and the patient is not legally competent to give an informed consent and/or a person legally authorized to consent on behalf of the patient is not readily available, his consent to required treatment will be implied. WASH. REV. CODE §7.70.050 (2008).

A dental hygienist's duty to disclose information generally requires disclosure of the following: (1) the nature of the patient's condition or diagnosis; (2) the nature and purpose of proposed treatment; (3) the risks, consequences, and anticipated results of the proposed treatment; (4) the alternative feasible treatment; (5) the risks, consequences, and anticipated results of the alternative feasible treatment; and (6) the probable or possible consequences of accepting no treatment. The discussion of risks should include the nature and severity of the risk and the likelihood of its occurrence. For example, patients with active periodontal disease may have a claim for failure to obtain informed consent if they are not informed of the potential consequences of limiting care to the annual prophylactic treatment covered by their insurance plan.

A breach of duty to obtain informed consent generally is not sufficient to establish a claim of lack of informed consent if the breach was not the cause of an injury to the patient. To establish a causal link between the breach of duty and patient injury, both *injury causation* and decision causation must exist. Injury causation requires that the patient suffer an adverse consequence and that the cause of the injury be an undisclosed risk. Decision causation requires demonstrating that the patient would not have consented to treatment (or in the case of no treatment, the patient would have consented to treatment) had the disclosure been adequate.

Who can Give Informed Consent?   Competent adults are solely responsible for the determination of the health care services to which they are willing to consent. Informed consent to the treatment of an adult patient may be sought from an authorized person other than the patient only when the patient is incapable of consenting because of incompetency or incapacity. Guidance in determining who is an authorized person to consent to care for an incompetent or incapacitated adult should be sought from statutory law, for example:

Informed consent—Persons authorized to provide for patients who are not competent—Priority. (1) Informed consent for health care for a patient who is not competent . . . to consent may be obtained from a person authorized to consent on behalf of such patient. (a) Persons authorized to provide informed consent to health care on behalf of a patient who is not competent to consent . . . shall be a member of one of the following classes of persons in the following order of priority: (i) The appointed guardian of the patient, if any; (ii) The individual, if any, to whom the patient has given a durable power of attorney that encompasses the authority to make health care decisions; (iii) The patient's spouse or state registered domestic partner; (iv) Children of the patient who are at least eighteen years of age; (v) Parents of the patient; and (vi) Adult brothers and sisters of the patient. (b) If the health care provider seeking informed consent for proposed health care of the patient who is not competent to consent . . . makes reasonable efforts to locate and secure authorization from a competent person in the first or succeeding class and finds no such person available, authorization may be given by any person in the next class in the order of descending priority. However, no person under this section may provide informed consent to health care: (i) If a person of higher priority under this section has refused to give such authorization; or (ii) If there are two or more individuals in the same class and the decision is not unanimous among all available members of that class. (c) Before any person authorized to provide informed consent on behalf of a patient not competent to consent . . . exercises that authority, the person must first determine in good faith that that patient, if competent, would consent to the proposed health care. If such a determination cannot be made, the decision to consent to the proposed health care may be made only after determining that the proposed health care is in the patient's best interests. WASH. REV. STAT. §7.70.065 (2008).

Minor patients generally are unable to consent legally to health care. In most jurisdictions the age of majority is attained at the age of 18 years. Therefore consent to treatment of persons younger than 18 years generally should be sought from the minor's parents. Parents who are themselves minors typically are granted authority to consent to the health care needs of their children. Other exceptions to the requirement of parental consent for the treatment of minors are the treatment of a minor in an emergency, the treatment of a legally recognized *emancipated* or mature *minor* (i.e., a minor who is free from parental control), or other statutorily authorized treatment of a consenting minor.

Documentation of Informed Consent. Informed consent is a process of communication between a dental hygienist and patient in which the patient acquires adequate information to make an autonomous and informed decision regarding his or her treatment plan. Information must be effectively conveyed to the patient to ensure comprehension. To ensure patient comprehension, the dental hygienist must speak and write clearly, using lay terminology. In addition, patients must be given the opportunity to ask questions and receive adequate answers.

In general, consent does not need to be written to be valid. However, from a practical perspective, consent that is not written may be difficult to prove. Written documentation of consent may take the form of an entry in the patient record, a consent document that acknowledges the required disclosures were made and understood, or a consent form that delineates the required disclosures and acknowledges understanding. The type of procedure to be performed and the nature and severity of risk, as well as the likelihood of its occurrence, can be used as guides for the selection of the form of consent. The patient's implied consent, by his or her presence in the dental chair, may be adequate consent for the performance of a clinical examination with minimal risk. Documentation of consent in the patient record, dated and initialed by the patient, may be sufficient for routine dental hygiene procedures that are not a part of a comprehensive treatment plan. A comprehensive treatment plan can be reviewed with patients and verified in writing by them with an accompanying statement that acknowledges that they have been informed of their condition and consent to the plan of care. For high-risk procedures, such as surgery, the use of a comprehensive and individualized consent form is advisable.

An education isn't how much you have committed to memory, or even how much you know. It's being able to differentiate between what you know and what you don't.

ANATOLE FRANCE

Professional Malpractice

Not unlike informed consent, professional malpractice had its beginning in common law. However, many jurisdictions have codified the requirements of claims relating to health care.

Malpractice Defined. In general, dental *malpractice* is the failure of an oral health care provider to exercise the degree of care, skill, and learning expected of a reasonably prudent oral health care provider, in the class to which he or she belongs within the state, acting in the same or similar circumstances. Some states, such as Arizona, provide protection against malpractice actions to providers delivering care as volunteers and not for compensation.

A health professional . . . who provides medical or dental treatment within the scope of the health professional's certificate or license at a nonprofit clinic where neither the professional nor the clinic receives compensation for any treatment provided at the clinic is not liable in a medical malpractice action, unless such health professional was grossly negligent. ARIZ. REV. STAT. §12-571 (A) (2008).

Malpractice may be established when a provider is found to have violated the standard of care. The standard of care can be established legislatively, administratively (see Oregon rules that follow), and through expert testimony.

Unacceptable patient care. The Board finds, using the criteria set forth in ORS 679.140(4), that a licensee engages in or permits the performance of unacceptable patient care if the licensee does or permits any person to: (1) Provide treatment which exposes a patient to risk of harm when equivalent or better treatment with less risk to the patient is available. (2) Fails to seek consultation whenever the welfare of a patient would be safeguarded or advanced by having recourse to those who have special skills, knowledge and experience; provided, however, that it is not a violation of this section to omit to seek consultation if other competent licensees in the same locality and in similar circumstances would not have sought such consultation. (3) Fail to provide or arrange for emergency treatment for a patient currently receiving treatment. (4) Fail to exercise supervision required by the Dental Practice Act over any person or permit any person to perform duties for which the person is not licensed or certified. (5) Render services which the licensee is not licensed to provide. (6) Fail to comply with ORS 453.605 to 453.755 or rules adopted pursuant thereto relating to the use of x-ray machines. (7) Fail to maintain patient records in accordance with OAR 818-012-0070. (8) Fail to provide goods or services in a reasonable period of time which are due to a patient pursuant to a contract with the patient or a third party. (9) Attempt to perform procedures which the licensee is not capable of performing due to physical or mental disability. (10) Perform any procedure for which the patient or patient's guardian has not previously given informed consent provided, however, that in an emergency situation, if the patient is a minor whose guardian is unavailable or the patient is unable to respond, a licensee may render treatment in a reasonable manner according to community standards. (11) Use the behavior management technique of Hand Over Mouth (HOM) without first obtaining informed consent for the use of the technique. (12) Use the behavior management technique of Hand Over Mouth Airway Restrictions (HOMAR) on any patient. OR. ADMIN. R. §818-012-0010 (2008).

Dental hygienists violate the standard of care when they injure a patient by not using the care, knowledge, skill, and ability possessed by other dental hygienists. For example, a dental hygienist would violate the standard of care if he or she failed to obtain a comprehensive health history on a patient before performing periodontal therapy. The dental hygienist may commit malpractice if this violation of the standard of care results in injury to the patient. The standard of care for dental hygiene includes responsibilities in patient assessment, treatment planning, treatment, patient education, and evaluation.

Shared Responsibility.   Health care injuries may be the result of both the provider's failure to meet the standard of care and the patient's failure to comply with the treatment plan. In such situations, the responsibility for the injury is shared by the patient and recognized as *contributory negligence.* Responsibility for health care injuries also may be shared between the provider and employer. The legal doctrine of "respondeat superior" stands for the proposition that employers act through their employees or agents and are therefore responsible for the negligent acts of their employees or agents. Therefore the dentist is not uncommonly a sole or joint defendant in cases of health care injury resulting from care delivered by a dental hygienist.

Education is the leading of human souls to what is best, and making what is best out of them.

JOHN RUSKIN

Statute of Limitations.   A *statute of limitations* is a statutory provision that limits the period within which an injured party can file a legal action. The purpose of these time limitations is to protect against stale claims that will be difficult to judge because of limited documentation and undependable recollection of events. Statutes of limitations for health care injury or malpractice actions vary by state; however, they usually are in the range of 2 to 4 years from the date of the alleged act, omission, neglect, or occurrence. Given that some injuries are not known at the time of their occurrence, a statute of limitations also provides for a period (1 to 2 years) for filing an action after discovery of an injury (see Utah statute that follows). For injuries to minors, the statute of limitations is tolled until they reach the age of majority.

> Statute of limitations—Exceptions—Application. (1) A malpractice action against a health care provider shall be commenced within two years after the plaintiff or patient discovers, or through the use of reasonable diligence should have discovered the injury, whichever first occurs, but not to exceed

four years after the date of the alleged act, omission, neglect or occurrence .UTAH CODE ANN. §78B-3-404 (1) (2008).

Reporting Requirements.   Some states, such as Arizona and Oklahoma, require that malpractice settlements and judgments against dental hygienists be reported to the state health profession regulatory board.

> If a medical malpractice action . . . is settled or a court enters a monetary judgment: 1. The professional liability insurers shall provide the defendant's health profession regulatory board with all information required to be filed with the national practitioner data bank . . . 2. The plaintiff's attorney shall provide the defendant's health profession regulatory board . . . with the notice required under subsection B of this section, a copy of the complaint and a copy of either the agreed terms of settlement or the judgment. The attorney shall provide this notice and these documents within thirty days after a settlement is reached or a judgment is entered. ARIZ. REV. STAT. §12-570 (A) (2008).
>
> Whenever a claim of personal injury is made against any practitioner of the healing arts or a licensed hospital, a report shall be made to the appropriate licensing board or agency by the liability insurer of such practitioner or hospital within sixty (60) days after receipt of information that a claim is being made. In the event that such claim is made against a party not insured, the report shall be made by the party . . . And whenever such claim or suit is concluded, the disposition shall be reported to the appropriate board or agency promptly. OKLA. STAT. TIT. 76 §17 (2008).

Such notice may then serve as cause for an investigation by the regulatory board regarding the professional's practice, for example:

> On receipt of a malpractice report and a copy of a malpractice complaint as provided in "12-570, the health profession regulatory board shall initiate an investigation into the matter to determine if the licensee is in violation of the statutes or rules governing licensure. ARIZ. REV. STAT. §32-3203 (2008).

Breach of Contract

The most common **breach of contract** claim associated with health care injuries is that the health care provider promised the patient that the injury suffered would not occur. For example, statements indicating that a proposed procedure will take care of "someone's troubles" and that there is "nothing much to the procedure" may represent promises that cannot be kept. Health care providers are not expected to be guarantors of health care outcomes. Therefore the dental hygienist should be careful not to make statements that a patient may interpret as a guarantee of outcome.

▨ Summary

The dental hygienist–patient relationship is a two-sided relationship with rights and responsibilities on each side. As a health care professional, the dental hygienist has an ethical and legal obligation to uphold the standards of the profession and avoid injury to the patient. When injury that should have been avoided does occur, the legal system is designed to provide retribution and compensation to the patient and society. Dental hygienists are responsible for understanding their legal obligations. This chapter provides a general overview of the legal context of the dental hygienist–patient relationship. Dental hygienists are encouraged to seek legal counsel when specific issues of concern arise.

CHAPTER 9

Dental Hygienist–Dentist–Employer Relationship

CHERYL A. CAMERON
AND PAMELA ZARKOWSKI

LEARNING OUTCOMES

- Describe the legal parameters of the employer-employee relationship and state the two general categories of employment.
- Identify the recommended strategies for preparing for a dental hygiene employment interview.
- List the items that can and cannot legally be asked during the application and interview process for a dental hygiene position.
- Describe the federal laws prohibiting discrimination and protecting worker safety.
- Explain the concepts of sexual harassment and hostile work environment in the dental practice setting.

KEY TERMS

civil rights
discrimination
employment
Equal Employment
  Opportunity
  Commission

federal laws
harassment
quid pro quo
sexual harassment

In most practice settings the dental hygienist will work as an employee for an employing dentist. As an employee, the dental hygienist must understand the legal parameters of the employer-employee relationship. The interests of employees are protected by numerous federal and state laws. Familiarity with these laws may help ensure a safe, productive, and professionally rewarding work environment for the dental hygienist.

The dental hygienist is an integral member of a dental practice and deserves to be treated with respect, dignity, and professionalism. Dental hygienists, together with the practices in which they are employed, will prosper when they are recognized for their professional contributions and acknowledged as valued members of a team. Compliance with federal and state employment laws is one way for an employer to give dental hygienists the professional recognition they deserve.

Although a dentist, as an employer, should be familiar with and comply with legal employment obligations, uninformed and unintentional violations can occur. Questions, potential oversights, and unintentional violations should be brought to the attention of the employer for resolution. However, when this does not result in satisfactory resolution and a dental hygienist suspects that his or her employment rights have been violated, an attorney or appropriate agency should be contacted for guidance and possible legal resolution. Such action should be viewed as the ethical and professional obligation of a dental hygienist.

Seeking and Obtaining Employment

When seeking employment, a dental hygienist may explore a number of different forums. Dental hygiene positions frequently are announced in classified advertisements in local newspapers and professional publications, such as newsletters and journals. Dental hygiene job placement services, which may be advertised in professional newsletters or telephone directories, are another source for identifying available positions. Word of mouth and networking with fellow professionals at meetings, continuing education programs, and community service events also can be a valuable mechanism for finding well-suited employment opportunities. The Internet also has made electronic posting of positions a viable means of finding available positions. Formal job announcements generally indicate the application procedure and provide details regarding the preferred mode of contact (telephone or in-person) and resume submission.

The selection process generally includes an interview with the employer. The interview may be limited to a question-and-answer period, or it may include a working interview, which provides an opportunity for the employer to assess the applicant's professional competence. When preparing for an interview, the dental hygienist should consider the following strategies:

- Prepare a concise, accurate, and professional resume that highlights educational background, employment history, and professional experiences, such as association membership, presentations, and honors.
- Obtain a job description and develop questions concerning practice philosophies and protocols, referral strategies, documentation guidelines, performance evaluation, and other pertinent information.
- Anticipate questions and plan responses to inquiries about career goals, professional skills and judgment, commitment to lifelong learning, and potential contributions to the practice.
- Be familiar with proper and improper employment inquiries during the interview process.

Limitations exist regarding the questions that may legally be asked during the hiring process. The following list provides examples of permissible inquiries during the application and interview process:

- Full name and any different names necessary to verify employment history
- Date of birth
- Length of residency in a particular state or city
- Name of relatives already employed by the employer
- Ability to perform the duties of the position with or without accommodation
- Ability to meet specified work schedules and attendance requirements
- U.S. citizenship or legal residency status
- Languages that can fluently be spoken and written
- Educational and employment history
- Criminal conviction history
- Emergency contact

The application and interview process is intended to support the selection of an applicant who is able to perform the functions of the available position. Questions are classified as impermissible when the information sought could be used in a discriminatory manner and is irrelevant in terms of assessing an applicant's qualifications for a position. However, once a hiring decision is made, certain additional information may be necessary for personnel records and employee benefit programs. The following list provides examples of inquiries not permitted during the application or interview process:

- Original name when changed by court order or marriage
- Marital status or related questions
- Number of children and their ages or related questions
- Gender
- National origin, ancestry, and descent
- Religion
- Race or color of skin
- Height and weight
- Disability status
- Arrest record
- Required list of affiliations and memberships
- Garnishment of wages

During the application and interview process, applicants should be cautious not to offer information voluntarily that cannot be solicited legally by the employer. Although a dental hygienist who is the proud mother of two fabulous children might be inclined to comment on her children after noticing pictures of the employer's children on his desk, she should think twice. A discussion of her children could raise concerns about child care arrangements and the impact of sick children on the employee's attendance record. Enough time exists to develop a personal relationship with the employer and other employees after the hiring decision is complete.

There is a big difference between what we have a right to do and what is right to do.

JUSTICE POTTER STUART

Employment Relationship

A dental hygienist can be employed within two general categories of **employment:** (1) at will and (2) term. The at will category is best described as employment with an indefinite duration. This means that the employment relationship can be terminated at the will of either the employer or employee for any or no reason. A dentist can inform a dental hygienist at the end of a work day that his or her employment in the office is terminated, effective immediately. Termination decisions customarily are accompanied by notice (e.g., 2 weeks before the end of the employment relationship) or severance pay. However, the termination of an at will employment relationship can legally occur without notice, severance pay, or a statement of cause as long as it is not made for a discriminatory reason.

The term *category* is best described as employment with a definite duration. For example, a dental hygienist may sign an employment contract for a period of 12 months. An employment contract generally has language that specifies the conditions under which the employment relationship can be terminated before the completion of the duration. The legal term for these conditions is *just cause.* The employment relationship cannot be terminated without breaching the contract unless just cause exists, which is a specified (i.e., contractually agreed upon) and nondiscriminatory reason for termination.

Employment Laws

Many federal and state employment laws are designed to protect the interests of employees and employers. Although the employer may have an obligation to inform employees of various state and *federal laws,* dental hygienists should be independently familiar with and know how to access additional information about their rights as employees.

Federal Laws Prohibiting Discrimination

Title VII of the Civil Rights Act of 1964. Title VII of the *Civil Rights* Act of 1964, 42 U.S.C.§§2000e et seq. (2008), is a federal law that protects against *discrimination* on the basis of race, color, religion, sex, or national origin. This act applies to employers with 15 or more employees. Discrimination is prohibited in any employment action including, but not limited to, hiring and firing, compensation and salary raises, promotions, fringe benefits, and retirement plans.

The Pregnancy Discrimination Act was an amendment to Title VII of the Civil Rights Act of 1964, 42 U.S.C. §2000e(k) (2008). This amendment prohibits employment discrimination on the basis of pregnancy, childbirth, or related medical conditions. An employer cannot refuse to hire a qualified applicant on the basis of pregnancy. An employer cannot treat pregnancy-related conditions differently by requesting that only pregnant employees undergo medical evaluation regarding ability to work. If an employer requires that all employees with a medical condition undergo medical evaluation to establish ability to work, then a pregnant employee can be required to comply with the same procedure (e.g., providing a statement from a health care provider documenting need for leave). If a temporary inability to work occurs, the pregnant employee must be treated like any other temporarily disabled employee in terms of available options, such as leave or leave without pay. An employer cannot have a policy that prohibits an employee from returning to work for a predetermined time after childbirth. Health insurance coverage provided by an employer must cover expenses for pregnancy-related conditions, with the exception of abortions unless the life of the mother would be endangered if the fetus were carried to term, on the same basis as costs for other medical conditions. Pregnancy benefits cannot be limited to married employees (e.g., 29 CFR §1604.10 [2008]).

> *We make a living by what we get; we make a life by what we give.*
>
> SIR WINSTON CHURCHILL

Equal Pay Act of 1963. The Equal Pay Act of 1963, 29 U.S.C. §206(d) (2008), is a federal law that protects men and women who perform substantially equal work in the same establishment from sex-based wage discrimination. An employer cannot reduce the wages of either a man or woman to equalize pay inequities (e.g., 29 CFR §§1620 [2008]).

Age Discrimination in Employment Act of 1967. The Age Discrimination in Employment Act of 1967, 29 U.S.C. §§621-634 (2008), is a federal law that prohibits discrimination based on age against any employee or applicant for employment who is at least 40 years old. The act applies to employers with 20 or more employees, including state and local government. Examples of age discrimination include a job advertisement that indicates age preferences and denial or cessation of benefits to older employees (e.g., 29 CFR §§1625 [2008]).

Americans with Disabilities Act of 1990. The Americans with Disabilities Act of 1990 42 U.S.C. §§12101 et seq. (2008) is a federal law that prohibits discrimination against qualified individuals with disabilities. This law applies to employers with 15 or more employees. An individual with a disability is defined as a person who has a physical or mental impairment that substantially limits one or more major life activities. Physical impairments include any physiologic disorder, condition, cosmetic disfigurement, or anatomic loss affecting one or more of the following body systems: neuro-logic, musculoskeletal, special sense organs, respiratory (including speech organs), cardiovascular, reproductive, digestive, genitourinary, hemic and lymphatic, skin, and endocrine. Mental impairments include any mental or psychological disorder, such as mental retardation, organic brain syndrome, emotional or mental illness, and specific learning disabilities. Major life activities include walking, breathing, seeing, hearing, speaking, learning, and working. The inability to perform a single, particular job does not constitute a substantial limitation in the major life activity of working. Examples of impairments that can limit major life activities include multiple sclerosis, asthma, diabetes, osteoporosis, bipolar disorder, dyslexia, and human immunodeficiency virus (HIV) infection. Although a history of drug addiction is recognized as an impairment, individuals currently using illegal drugs are not protected by this act.

Disabled individuals can qualify for protection under the Americans with Disabilities Act if they satisfy skill, experience, education, and other job-related requirements of a position and also can perform the job with or without reasonable accommodation. Employers are required to provide reasonable accommodation to a qualified disabled employee or job applicant. Three categories of reasonable accommodation exist: (1) changes to the job application process, (2) changes to the work environment or the way a job is usually performed, and (3) changes that allow an employee with a disability to enjoy equal benefits and privileges of employment. Reasonable accommodation can include making existing facilities accessible, modifying schedules, or modifying equipment. For example, an office manager with hearing loss may need telephones equipped with sound amplification to function in the position. Reasonable accommodations do not include modifications that would cause an undue hardship to the employer.

Before making a job offer to a potential employee, an employer cannot ask an applicant about the existence, nature, or severity of a disability. However, the employer can and should inform the applicant of the essential functions of the position and inquire whether the applicant is able, with or without accommodation, to perform those job functions (e.g., 29 CFR §§1630 [2008]).

Uniformed Services Employment and Reemployment Rights Act of 1994. The Uniformed Services Employment and Reemployment Rights Act of 1994, 38 U.S.C. §§4301-4334 (2008), is a federal law that protects civilian job rights and benefits for veterans and members of Reserve components. This law is administered and enforced by the Department of Labor (www.dol.gov/vets/programs/userra/).

State Laws Prohibiting Discrimination

States may enact laws that extend the provisions of the federal laws against employment discrimination. Such state laws may extend the reach of the non-discrimination provisions (e.g., redefining "employer" to require fewer employees to be bound by the employment discrimination laws). For instance, the "law against discrimination" in the state of Washington, WASH. REV. CODE §49.60.040(3) (2008), defines an employer as any person who employs eight or more persons. Other state laws may extend the scope of protections (e.g., redefining the term "disability" to include a broader scope of conditions or extending the protected categories). For instance, the "law against discrimination" in the state of Washington, WASH. REV. CODE §49.60.180 (2008), prohibits employment discrimination against any person because of "the presence of any sensory, mental, or physical disability" and extends the protected categories to include "sexual orientation." Still other laws extend the nature of available remedies.

Enforcement of Laws Prohibiting Discrimination

The *Equal Employment Opportunity Commission* (EEOC) enforces the federal laws against discrimination in the employment setting. The EEOC has several field offices to assist individuals who believe they are the subjects of a violation of a federal law. Individuals who believe they have experienced a violation of their employment rights may file a charge of discrimination with the EEOC. The process is not complicated; however, specific guidelines and time frames must be followed (see the box on page 147). It is unlawful for an employer to retaliate or take adverse action (e.g., by refusing to hire, denying job benefits, or making threats) against an employee who opposes any violations of the employment discrimination laws (e.g., refuses to answer impermissible interview questions, suggests treatment is unequal on the basis of disability, or complains to a co-worker about sexually harassing behavior) or files a complaint with the EEOC (42 U.S.C. §2000e-3 2008). More details about the federal laws prohibiting employment discrimination can be obtained at the EEOC website at www.eeoc.gov.

Individuals also may file complaints with their state commission (e.g., human rights commission or civil rights office) when concern exists that state laws are being violated.

Other Laws Providing Employee Protections

Family Medical Leave Act of 1993. The Family Medical Leave Act of 1993 (FMLA), 29 U.S.C. §§2601-2654 (2008), is a federal law that makes available medically necessary leave to qualified employees.

FILING AN EEOC CLAIM FOR DISCRIMINATION

- Any individual who believes that his or her employment rights have been violated may file a charge of discrimination with the EEOC.
- A charge may be filed personally or by mail to the nearest EEOC office. An individual interested in filing a claim can consult the local telephone directory (U.S. government listing) or call 800-669-4000 or 800-669-6820 (TTY) to locate the nearest office. (Access www. eeoc.gov/offices.html to contact your local field office.)
- When filing a complaint, the information required includes (1) the complaining party's name, address, and telephone number; (2) the name, address, and telephone number of the person or agency alleged to have discriminated and the number of employees at the workplace; and (3) a short description of the alleged violation.
- Strict time limits exist within which charges must be filed. A charge must be filed with the EEOC within 180 days from the date of the alleged violation. Exceptions exist, but contacting the EEOC promptly when discrimination is suspected is best.
- Once a charge has been filed, the employer is notified. Resolution of the charges is determined based on a review of the facts by the EEOC.
- Resolution of the charge may involve various courses of action. An attempt may be made to remedy the discrimination. Remedies may include, but are not limited to, back pay, promotion, reinstatement, hiring, front pay, reasonable accommodation, or other actions that would make the complainant "whole." If the EEOC's attempt to conciliate a remedy is unsuccessful, legal action may be available.
- Additional information may be obtained from the U.S. Equal Employment Opportunity Commission at 1801 L Street NW, Washington, DC 20507; 202-663-4900 or 202-633-4494 (TTY).
- Publications are available that advise employees of their equal opportunity employment rights. To obtain this information, contact the EEOC at www.eeoc.gov/publications.html; 800-669-3362 or 800-800-3302 (TTY); 301-206-9789 (fax).

The FMLA applies to public and private employers with 50 or more employees. To be eligible, an employee must have worked for the employer for 12 months and worked at least 1250 hours over the previous 12 months. Under the FMLA an employer must grant an eligible employee up to 12 weeks of unpaid leave during a 12-month period for the following reasons:

- Birth and care of a newborn child
- Placement of a child for adoption or foster care
- Provision of care for an immediate family member (spouse, child, or parent) with a serious health condition
- Serious health condition that makes an employee unable to perform the function of his or her position
- Any qualifying exigency arising out of the fact that a family member (spouse, child, or parent) is on active duty in the Armed Forces in support of a contingency operation

An extended period of leave of a total of 26 work weeks, for a single 12-month period, may be available to an employee who is the spouse, child, parent, or next of kin of a covered service member requiring care.

In some circumstances the FMLA permits leaves to be taken intermittently, such as taking leave in blocks of time or reducing a normal daily or weekly schedule. When possible, employees should give their employer 30 days notice before beginning an FMLA leave. During an approved FMLA leave, an employer must maintain the insurance benefits provided as a part of the employment relationship. Upon return to employment, an employee is required to be restored to his or her original position or to an equivalent position with equivalent pay, benefits, and other terms and conditions of employment. More details on FMLA can be obtained at the U.S. Department of Labor website at www.dol.gov/compliance/laws/comp-fmla.htm.

States may enact laws that extend the provisions of the FMLA. For example, domestic violence leave is available in the state of Washington to victims of domestic violation, sexual assault, and stalking to seek legal or law enforcement assistance; to seek treatment by a health care provider for physical or mental injuries; to obtain services from a domestic violence shelter, rape crisis center, or other social services programs; or to participate in safety planning activities (Domestic Violence Leave, ch. 49.76 WASH. REV. CODE).

Occupational Safety and Health Act of 1970.   The Occupational Safety and Health Act (OSHA) of 1970, 29 U.S.C. §§651-678 (2008), is a federal law intended to ensure safe and healthful working conditions for employees. The law places responsibility on employers and employees to comply with established standards and training requirements intended to minimize the number of personal injuries and illnesses that arise out of employment. In general, employers are obligated to provide a place of employment free from recognized hazards that may cause serious physical harm to their employees. For example, OSHA standards require that dentist employers provide personal protective equipment in the dental office to minimize the hazards associated with contact with blood-borne pathogens. Employees, in turn, are obligated to comply with OSHA standards applicable to their scope of employment. State laws also may be enacted that equal or exceed the requirements imposed by OSHA. For example, the state of Washington enacted the Washington Industrial Safety and Health Act, ch. 49.17 WASH. REV. CODE. See www.osha.gov/dcsp/osp/index.html for more information on state-approved plans. More details on OSHA can be obtained at the OSHA website at www.osha.gov.

State workers' compensation provisions provide relief for employees who are injured while acting in the course of their employment. Dental hygienists who are injured at work should notify their employer dentist of the injury and seek assistance in complying with the requirements of the workers' compensation program. Quick access to government programs can be found on the Internet. The home pages of the state government websites can be found at www.usa.gov/Agencies/State_and_Territories.shtml.

> *C*ourage is not simply one of the virtues, but the form of every virtue at the testing point.
>
> C.S. LEWIS

Sexual Harassment

The dental office environment, like many employment settings, provides opportunities for frequent interaction between male and female colleagues. Multiple levels of interactions occur, including employer-employee, employee-employee, and employer/employee-patient/client. Each of these levels of interaction provides an opportunity for inappropriate behavior.

Oral health care providers work in close contact with their colleagues and patients. Dental hygienists must be aware of behaviors that could be interpreted as *sexual harassment.* Sexual harassment is an illegal activity. Dental hygienists may be targeted for inappropriate discussions, behaviors, or pictures from employers, colleagues, patients, or vendors visiting an employment setting. A harasser may be male or female, and an accuser may be of the same or different gender.

Sexual harassment is a form of discrimination that violates Title VII of the Civil Rights Act of 1964. Federal regulations define sexual harassment as unwelcome sexual advances, requests for sexual favors, and other verbal or physical conduct of a sexual nature when submission to such conduct is made either explicitly or implicitly a term or condition of an individual's employment; submission to or rejection of such conduct by an individual is used as the basis for employment decisions affecting such individual; or such conduct has the purpose or effect of unreasonably interfering with an individual's work performance or creating an intimidating, hostile, or offensive working environment.

Categories of Harassing Behavior

Sexually harassing behavior falls into two categories: (1) quid pro quo and (2) hostile environment. **Quid pro quo** means "something for something." Quid pro quo **harassment** occurs when (1) an individual's submission to or rejection of sexual advances or conduct of a sexual nature is used as the basis for employment decisions affecting the individual, or (2) the individual's submission to such conduct is made a term or condition of employment. To be actionable, an individual must be subjected to unwelcome harassment. Unwelcome harassment occurs when harassment is based on sex and when the individual's reaction to the harassment affects tangible aspects of his or her compensation, terms, conditions, or privileges of employment. An employer who requests a sexual favor from an employee in exchange for a raise or monetary bonus may be guilty of quid pro quo harassment.

A hostile environment occurs when any type of unwelcome sexual behavior creates an offensive or hostile environment. The harassment does not need to result in tangible or economic job consequences, such as the loss of pay or promotion opportunities. To prove a hostile environment, the harassment must be proven to have been unwelcome. The harassment must be sufficiently severe or pervasive as to create an abusive working environment. An important criterion is that the employer had actual knowledge or constructive knowledge of the hostile environment but took no remedial or prompt action. Constructive knowledge is a legal term that means that employer, under the circumstances, should have known about the hostile work environment. An environment is hostile if a reasonable person would find the environment hostile or abusive and the victim subjectively perceives the environment to be abusive. Examples of behaviors that may create a hostile work environment if sufficiently severe or pervasive include the following:

- Unsolicited or unwelcome flirtations or propositions
- Conversation with a sexual content
- Suggestive comments about one's appearance

- Unwanted touching
- Display of sexually suggestive objects or pictures
- Intrusive questions about the employee's personal life
- Descriptions of the harasser's sexual experiences
- Use of diminutive terms, such as "honey"

Protection for the Dental Hygienist

Sexual harassment often is discussed in terms of a "power" relationship, meaning one individual has authority over another. An individual, such as an employer or professor, has the power to determine a promotion or a grade. Hostile environments may be created when a person of authority takes advantage of that authority and requests activity of a sexual nature. Because the individual is the person of authority, the target may be fearful of not complying. Power or authority does not allow an individual to violate another person's rights. An employer, colleague, or patient may be unaware that his or her behavior is offensive. A dental office may develop an office manual that outlines appropriate and inappropriate behavior and consequences for failure to fulfill specific guidelines. However, whether or not an office policy exists, if dental hygienists are subjected to behaviors that create a hostile environment steps can be taken legally and personally to protect them.

If a dental hygienist is sexually harassed on the job, he or she should do the following:

- Say *no* clearly. Make it clear to the harasser that attentions are unwanted and that his or her behavior is offensive. Name the specific behavior. Write a memo to the harasser asking that the behavior stop; always keep a copy.
- Hold the harasser accountable for his or her actions. Do not make excuses and do not pretend the incident never occurred. Let people know what happened. Privacy protects harassers; visibility undermines them.
- Document the harassment. Write down each incident, including date, time, and place. Detail what happened, including response. Keep a copy at home.
- Document your work. Keep a copy of performance evaluations and memos that indicate the quality of your performance. The harasser, if an employer or supervisor, may question your job performance to justify his or her behavior.
- Look for other individuals in the work environment who also may have been targeted by the harasser or who witnessed the offensive behavior.

- Explore office policy and protocol. Review the office manual or grievance procedures outlined in the employee handbook.
- File a complaint. If a legal remedy is necessary, contact a state discriminatory agency or the federal EEOC. The federal agency covers workplaces of 15 or more employees; however, individual state law may protect the dental hygienist if he or she is employed in a workplace with fewer staff members.
- Contact an attorney. If a discussion of the situation is warranted, an attorney specializing in employment discrimination is advised.

The quality of a person's life is in direct proportion to their commitment to excellence, regardless of their field of endeavor.

VINCE LOMBARDI

Summary

Because of the importance of commerce in society, employment is highly regulated by federal and state government. Such regulation is intended to protect the welfare of society by safeguarding the individual interests of employees. Dental hygienists are likely to work as employees during the course of their career. They must be informed of federal and state employment laws and act to ensure that their rights and responsibilities are upheld.

CHAPTER 10

Risk Management

PHYLLIS L. BEEMSTERBOER,
CHERYL A. CAMERON,
AND PAMELA ZARKOWSKI

LEARNING OUTCOMES

- Describe the concept of risk management and its place in the practice of dental hygiene.
- Identify the strategies that can be used to identify and reduce risk in the dental practice.
- List the elements of a good dental record and describe practices that should be considered in maintaining dental documentation.
- Discuss the role of verbal and nonverbal communication in the patient-provider relationship.
- Explain how dental hygienists should manage their own professional credentials and competency.

KEY TERMS

dental record
incident reporting
quality assessment

quality improvement
risk identification

The primary goal of the dental hygienist is to provide care to patients that promotes the prevention of oral disease and the maintenance of oral health. However, as with most goals, the delivery of dental hygiene services brings with it the potential for unanticipated and untoward outcomes. For example, periodontal therapy is intended to help prevent the progression of disease and restore the patient to a state of oral health. Retention of a broken curette tip in a subgingival furcation certainly would be an untoward outcome of periodontal debridement. Pain management through local anesthesia is intended to maximize a patient's comfort during the delivery of services. An adverse reaction to local anesthetic unquestionably would be a disturbing and unwanted event.

> *Destiny is not a matter of chance; it is a matter of choice. It is not a thing to be waited for; it is a thing to be achieved.*
>
> JEREMY KITSON

The dental hygienist must anticipate potential untoward outcomes and implement strategies to minimize their occurrence. *Risk management* is a term that describes a philosophy of **risk identification** and system of injury prevention. The term also is applied to other areas of private and public business but is most frequently used in health care. Management, as part of the term, means that once risk is identified, it is measured for the seriousness of the potential outcome and the likelihood of its occurrence. A strategy is then created to handle the risk in such a way as to minimize it or, in some cases, to eliminate it altogether. For example, in a hospital setting providing heart or lung transplants may be a desirable service, but it may be deemed too high of a risk because of the cost and mortality rate. A general dental practice may not provide complex oral surgery procedures for patients because the clinicians have determined that extensive risk factors are associated with those procedures. The liability associated with complex oral surgery procedures may be too significant, thus making the risk greater than the benefit to the dental practice. In these cases the risk management strategy is the removal of a procedure from the scope of care delivery. Eliminating a high-risk procedure from the scope of practice is not always possible or desirable. In such cases a risk management strategy should be implemented to control the risk.

Risk Identification

The development of well-targeted procedures for minimizing adverse outcomes requires an awareness of the most frequently occurring negative incidents. Familiarity with the professional literature can support the dental hygienist in anticipating possible undesired outcomes. Another approach, which focuses on a specific practice, is a system of *incident reporting.* Such a system requires that the members of the dental team complete a report for all accidents or unusual incidents. Reporting should include patient care problems, patient management issues, and patient complaints. Such a report should focus on the reporting of facts rather than subjective assessments and provide details of the event, including who, what, where, when, and why. These reports should not be retained in the patient record, but rather filed in a risk management portfolio. An incident reporting system permits the systematic tracking of adverse events. A clear understanding of the risk exposure of a practice provides an opportunity for targeted problem solving.

Another strategy for risk identification is the implementation of a *quality improvement* program. The purpose of a quality improvement program is to assess the patient care delivery system systematically and continuously through the collection and analysis of reliable information. The quality improvement process is an ongoing evaluation system that focuses on patterns of behavior rather than on isolated instances of behavior (i.e., incident reporting). It is a mechanism for assessing the quality of care and implementing and evaluating changes in the patient care delivery system to maintain or improve the quality of care. A quality improvement program should include three dimensions of health care delivery: structure, process, and outcome (Box 10-1). The structure dimension considers physical plant factors, such as facilities and equipment. The process dimension considers patient care issues, such as diagnosis, sequence of care, and technical skill. The outcomes dimension considers the result of care, such as improvements in oral health or overall health.

Growth requires us to become intimate with what is foreign.

ALICE WALKER

The first step in a quality improvement process is the assessment of quality in one or more of the dimensions of health care delivery. This *quality*

BOX 10-1

Dimensions of Quality Improvement

STRUCTURE	PROCESS	OUTCOMES
Facilities	Diagnoses	Oral health improvement
Equipment	Sequence of care	
Organization	Appropriateness of care	General health improvement
Administration	Technical skill	
Personnel	Timeliness of care	
Dental records		

assessment must be performed systematically and include designing a study, collecting data, analyzing data, reporting results, and responding to results. The next step is to design and implement strategies intended to improve the quality of the health care delivery system. The final step is to evaluate the effect of these strategies in improving and maintaining quality. Quality improvement is a continuous, cyclic process of assessment, planning, implementation, and evaluation.

In response to a concern that the dental hygiene instruments used in a practice may be at high risk for breakage, a study could be designed to assess the quality of the instruments. For example, on a given day a random sample of dental hygiene instruments may be selected for assessment. A reporting form that includes specific criteria, such as instrument type, tip length, tip width, and sharpness, could be designed for assessing the performance status of each instrument. The outcomes of this study could then be used to determine whether unusable instruments are inappropriately included in the instrument setups used by the dental hygienist. Depending on the results, modifications can be made to the instrument maintenance program to help ensure that the dental hygiene instrument trays are appropriately equipped. This quality improvement program focuses on the structure dimension of dental hygiene care.

A protocol designed to ensure compliance with the practice's health history policy is an example of a quality improvement program that focuses on the process dimension of care. A random sample of the records of patients who received periodontal maintenance therapy in a given period could be audited for compliance. An audit form should be designed to include the criteria that represent policy compliance (e.g., blood pressure documented, patient signature, dated entries). The results of the assessment can be used to acknowledge and reinforce policy compliance or to design in-service education that will support future compliance.

The outcome dimension can be assessed through posttreatment studies that consider the effects of dental hygiene care (e.g., results of patient education programs and therapeutic interventions). Patient satisfaction surveys are a valuable assessment tool for quality improvement. They permit a review of success from the patient's perspective and can include the structure dimension of care (e.g., Was the dental office clean and well maintained?), the dimension process (e.g., Did the dental hygienist communicate effectively?), and the outcome dimension (e.g., Has your daily home care improved?). Patient satisfaction surveys should be designed so that they gather the desired information and are easily completed. Survey participation can be encouraged by compensating patients with incentives, such as oral health care products, as a way of acknowledging the value of their time.

Risk Reduction

Two universally accepted strategies are used to minimize the risks associated with dental services: (1) good documentation and (2) careful communication in the care and treatment of the patient.

> *Every great mistake has a halfway moment when it can be recalled and perhaps remedied.*
>
> PEARL S. BUCK

Documentation

The foundation for good documentation in the dental office is the patient record. Documentation as part of the provision of oral health care services is important to protect the patient and the oral health care provider. The *dental record* is the comprehensive, ongoing file of assessment findings, treatment services rendered, dental outcomes, notations, and contacts with the patient. Each of the entries in the dental record should be signed and dated.

The record includes the baseline data gathered at the first encounter as well as a chronologic history of subsequent patient visits. If any type of legal action is initiated, the dental record, which contains the details of patient care, is the vital document that can (or cannot) protect the oral health care provider. All patient contacts should be recorded, including cancellations, messages left with the front desk, and calls for information. The fundamental requirement for effective and meaningful dental records is the implementation of a systematic process of accurate and complete documentation. The dental record should include the following:

- Personal data on the patient that must be updated routinely, including addresses, telephone numbers, contact information, and insurance payers.
- A health history, which should include information that has been collected and recorded in a systematic manner, with all conditions or areas of incomplete data noted and pursued. The type and amount of drugs the patient has taken must be recorded correctly and considered in dental treatment.
- A dental history, including information on previous treatments and the patient's response to those treatments.
- Care and treatment, including a careful recording of assessments performed, treatments rendered with informed consent, details of the conditions presented, medications and anesthetics provided, suggestions for postoperative care, and extent of patient education activities.
- Notes from conversations regarding the patient that are held with other health care professionals, or requests for consultations.

Comments about the patient encounter can be recorded in the dental record, but they must be related to the care of the patient and be stated in objective, professional, nonjudgmental terms. For example, a patient suspected of being under the influence of excessive alcohol consumption should be described according to the conditions observed, such as heavy odor of alcohol, slurred speech, or unsteadiness requiring assistance as opposed to a conclusive statement that the patient was drunk. If an entry is made in error, a single line should be drawn through the entry, followed by a note that an error was made. The correct information should then be recorded and the entry signed and dated.[1] When a correction is distanced from the error by intermediate entries, a notation should be made regarding the location of the error and its correction. The process of documentation should not be relegated to another staff person and should be completed in a timely manner after the patient visit. Delaying the entry may cause incomplete and inaccurate documentation. When documentation waits until the end of the day or after the dental hygienist has treated other patients, the risk of confusion is increased regarding which procedures were provided to which patient.

Abbreviations and professional jargon should be avoided unless a clear definition of terms is used within the dental practice that is readily documented. A simple note such as "prophy" is not appropriate because it does not convey what procedures were performed or how the patient responded to treatment and patient education. The following guidelines should be considered in maintaining the dental record:

- The dental record should be consistent for all patients. The office should develop an acceptable order of entries that best meets the needs of the practice. For example, a preprinted chart may be ordered that starts with patient identification and insurance information and proceeds to a medical and dental history; additional assessment data, such as intraoral and extraoral findings; radiographic records; treatment notes; consultation notes; and a financial/payment record.
- The dental team should be familiar with state laws regarding medical and dental records. State dental practice acts may dictate the information that must be included in a record and the length of time the record must be kept by the dental practice. Good risk management practice may call for keeping a dental record beyond the legally mandated retention date because dental records are the best defense in any legal action.
- Dental offices should develop guidelines for the order of treatment notes. In an office with multiple dental hygienists, all the hygienists should agree to a common format for treatment entry. This consistency assists in patient care and documents information for those who will provide subsequent treatment.
- The dental record should periodically be reviewed and updated. Health and dental history questions should be updated to reflect current general and dental health issues and trends.
- Entries should be clear, concise, legible. and permanent (e.g., black or blue permanent ballpoint ink).
- Errors should be corrected by an additional entry. For example, the care provider should write the phrase "Correction to entry of 9/6/08" or "Addition to entry of 9/6/08" as soon as possible after the error is identified. For paper records, the use of liquid correction fluid or correction tape to "white out" an entry should be avoided because this may be viewed as an attempt to hide information.
- Electronic record keeping is a common and acceptable method of maintaining patient information and should follow the general documentation guidelines. Steps must be in place to ensure that the record cannot be tampered with and that a valid signature is associated with each entry.

■ Commonly understood acronyms should be used so that all members of the office staff are familiar with the meaning of the term. Unusual or creative shorthand should not be used in dental documentation.

Risk management in record keeping is not limited to written entries. Documentation, broadly defined, includes radiographs, models, and photographs. The dental practice should maintain the quality of additional information gathered. Appropriate identification information, such as the patient's name, the current date, and the patient's chart number, should be marked on items such as models, radiographs, and photographs.

If patients terminate their relationship with a particular dental office, they may request that their dental records be forwarded to another dental health care practice. Patients have a legal right to a copy of their dental records (Health Insurance Portability and Accountability Act [HIPAA] 42 U.S.C. §§1320 et seq. [2008], 45 C.F.R. §164.524 [2007]). Patients must receive notice of these rights (45 C.F.R. §164.520 [2007]). A dental office may charge a patient a reasonable fee to duplicate the records and radiographs that will be forwarded. If a patient requests a record transfer, that request must be made in writing and dated, bear the patient's signature, identify the disclosing and receiving persons, specify the information to be disclosed, state an expiration date, and articulate the patient's right to revoke the authorization in writing (45 C.F.R. §164.508 [2007]).

A patient shares personal information with a dental hygienist or dentist with the understanding that the information will not be discussed or distributed inappropriately. All health care providers must recognize the importance of confidentiality and guard this special trust, which has both ethical and legal ramifications.

Listening is the shortest distance between two people.

UNKNOWN

Communication

Communication is the key to a successful, safe, and satisfying dental hygiene practice. The relationship that is established and that develops between the patient and the dental hygienist relies on verbal and nonverbal communication. Effective communication ensures that the needs of the patient and dental hygienist are clearly conveyed. Communication also is essential between the dentist employer, colleagues in the dental office, and other health care providers. The dental hygienist uses various levels of communication skills on a daily basis, constantly adapting, changing, and adjusting to the needs of patients and colleagues in the dental environment. The ultimate success of verbal communication depends on the way the material is presented, the attitude of the speaker, the tone and volume of voice, and the degree to which the dental hygienist and patient/colleague are able and ready to listen effectively.[2]

Lack of appropriate vocabulary and the use of jargon or words that are unfamiliar to the individual being spoken to are frequent complaints in the dental office. Clarity and a well-organized progression of ideas can help ensure an adequate level of understanding. This may require additional time, and the dental hygienist may need to stop periodically to check whether the receiving party comprehends the information being given. The attitude and tone with which the spoken words are presented also can have an impact on the effectiveness of the communication. Judgmental or negative attitudes and tone can influence the patient's response to the information or distract the patient from the educational message the hygienist is trying to convey.

Careful attention to the volume of the voice also is important. Volume should be adequate to ensure that the parties involved can hear what is being said without the information being overheard by uninvolved parties. Every patient wants to have the full and complete attention of the individual providing care, and many misunderstandings stem from the perception that the caregiver is not listening to the patient's issues. Purtilo and Haddad[2] recommend that the following strategies be used to improve the effectiveness of listening in a patient-provider interchange:

- Concentrate on central themes rather than isolated statements; listen in paragraphs.
- Listen with an open mind rather than focus on emotionally charged words.
- Summarize in your own mind what you have heard before speaking again.
- Clarify positions and statements before proceeding. Do not allow vague or incomplete ideas to go unchallenged.

After performing dental procedures, written instructions commonly are provided to the patient. This usually is done to reinforce verbal instruction. These written messages should be clear, concise, and accurate. Distribution of printed information, such as materials from the American Dental Association (ADA) or American Association of Periodontology (AAP), is quite acceptable, but these materials should be similar to the instructions provided, not contradictory or confusing. Providing an opportunity for questions and answers enhances patient understanding.

Nonverbal communication is as critical in a patient-provider interchange, as is the spoken word. This is especially true in the dental setting, where the patient often is unable to ask a question because of hands or instruments in the mouth. Facial expressions and gestures often communicate a great deal, and the dental hygienist must be sensitive to the messages sent through this avenue. Reading the patient's eyes is a common method for gauging a patient's reactions to diagnostic or treatment methods. Reassurance that a patient's response to a procedure is within the range of normal can be a welcome message, especially when dental hygiene treatments may be unfamiliar to them. Nonverbal communication is a two-way form of communication that warrants monitoring by the dental hygienist. Patients also receive communication, accurate or not, from the dental hygienists' nonverbal communication. For instance, frowns of concentration during treatment can be misunderstood as frowns of concern or criticism.

> *T*he greatest problem in communication is the illusion that it has been accomplished.
>
> GEORGE BERNARD SHAW

Changes in the demographics of the U.S. population have brought people from various lands and cultures into the dental setting. Health care providers must be sensitive to culture and ethnicity differences in the patients they treat.[3] What is a normal or expected practice in one country may be vastly different from what is done in the United States. Some of the differences among people are obvious, such as race or dress; others are much more difficult to ascertain. Most health care providers have been raised and educated among people like themselves and hold similar values and beliefs. Even a generational gap between a health care provider and an older patient can present some challenging issues of understanding. Treating patients with cultural differences is like treating any other patient; it must be done with understanding and respect. Cultural competence is an essential aspect of health care delivery. Learning about and being open to differences in cultures can help the dental hygienist provide sensitive and effective health care, honoring the autonomy of each person receiving dental hygiene services.

E-mail and other forms of electronic communication between patients and health care providers are becoming more common. Any electronic communication should comply with good practices for verbal and nonverbal communication. This communication must be clear, concise, and accurate. The "voice" of an electronic communication may be more easily misunderstood, so review messages carefully before sending to ensure they are professional, comprehendible, appropriately compassionate, and culturally sensitive.

When documenting aspects of the communication between dental hygienist and patient, the dental hygienist should ensure that the notations are factual and do not reflect a bias or subjective conclusion. If a direct quote from a patient is pertinent to the documentation, provide the quote with quotation marks. This allows interpretation of the patient's comments to be made by each health care provider.

> Success is not the key to happiness. Happiness is the key to success. If you love what you are doing, you will be successful.
>
> ALBERT SCHWEITZER

Individual Risk Management

The individual dental hygienist is responsible for managing his or her own professional competency and maintaining the appropriate credentials associated with being a licensed professional. Each dental hygienist must be familiar with the scope of practice allowed by the state dental practice act. If applicable, familiarity with the requirements for continuing education also is important. All continuing education courses should be carefully evaluated in terms of the quality of the information presented and the credentials of the presenters. Poor-quality continuing education that provides outdated or incorrect information may cause the practitioner to alter standard practices, putting the dental hygienist at risk. Belonging to a professional association, such as the American Dental Hygienist's Association (ADHA) and its related state and component societies, provides an additional source of continuing education and publications to keep the dental hygienist current. A dental hygienist also can become a member of other organizations, such as the Special Care Dentistry Association and the American Association of Public Health Dentists, or other groups that support a particular interest or focus. Professional dental groups as a course of business have publications and annual meetings that serve as sources of up-to-date information. Dental and dental hygiene education programs can be another source of up-to-date continuing education opportunities.

Most state practice acts require that any licensed dental health provider inform the monitoring agency of any address or name changes within a certain period. Renewal of a dental hygiene license usually is accomplished by paying a fee and providing documentation of continuing education. If a current cardiopulmonary resuscitation (CPR) card is a requirement for licensure renewal, the dental hygienist may need to offer proof of compliance in that area as well. Each dental hygienist should maintain a file of related professional documentation that includes licensure, liability insurance, and continuing education information.

A dental hygienist should consider other strategies to reduce individual risk. Maintaining a good working relationship with colleagues in the dental office is critical. Being respectful to patients and cautious about personal conversations, jokes, and inappropriate behavior that may be misinterpreted is also important. A dental hygienist should never provide treatment for which he or she is not qualified, educated, experienced, or licensed to perform.

Dental hygienists should carry adequate professional liability insurance and be familiar with the policy and its coverage, terms, and requirements. Understanding the nature of the coverage provided by a policy is essential. Claims-made coverage is limited to protection for allegations that arise from treatment rendered and reported while the policy is in force. Supplementation to claims-made coverage with tail coverage may be advisable; it preserves protection for claims made after the claims-made policy expires. Occurrence coverage extends protection to allegations arising from treatment rendered while the policy was in force even if the claim is reported after the policy has been cancelled. Policy terms to consider include the liability limits and deductibles that will apply. Many policies have restrictions or mandates for reporting if and when the hygienist is faced with a potential lawsuit. It also is advisable to contact an attorney for advice before entering into any binding agreement or when confronted with situations that have legal implications.

Summary

The dental hygienist has the ability to consider and apply numerous strategies that can identify and reduce the risk of unwanted consequences that may occur in dental hygiene practice. Risk management practices, established as a system or individually, can enhance the health and safety of the dental patient and support the ultimate goal of promoting oral health.

The road to happiness lies in two simple principles: find what it is that interests you and that you can do well, and when you find it put your whole soul into it—every bit of energy and ambition and natural ability you have.

JOHN D. ROCKEFELLER

REFERENCES

1 Pollack BR: *Dentist's risk management guide,* Ft. Lauderdale, FL, 1990, National Society of Dental Practitioners.
2 Purtilo R, Haddad A: *Health professional and patient interaction,* ed 7, Philadelphia, 2007, Saunders Elsevier.
3 Garcia RI: Addressing oral health disparities in diverse populations, *J Am Dent Assoc* 136:1210, 2005.

SECTION III

Simulations and Applications

Case Studies, Testlets, and Activities

Cases for Study and Discussion

The following cases are presented to allow the student of dental hygiene the opportunity to understand the types of ethical and legal dilemmas that may be encountered in the practice of dental hygiene.

An expert in dental and dental hygiene ethics has authored each case, and a wide variety of possible scenarios are presented for discussion and analysis. Some questions to stimulate thought and discussion are provided by each author. The ethical decision-making model presented in Chapter 6 can be applied in each of the cases.

Case-based ethics discussion is a common method used in ethics courses for dental and dental hygiene students. All the cases were designed to make the student consider the various aspects of the situation and, if desired, apply and follow the ethical decision-making model. The worksheet provided in Chapter 6 may be used to help structure the response to each case. This can be done as a solo assignment in a classroom setting, in small discussion groups, with an expert faculty panel, or in a continuing education environment with experienced dental hygienists.

CASE 1

Hygienist in the Middle

ALVIN B. ROSENBLUM
University of Southern California

A dental hygienist saw a patient for a routine scaling in the office of a general dentist. She found a periodontal problem that had not been noted previously in the patient's chart. She explained to the patient the existence of an abnormality and that she would talk about it with the dentist.

She communicated to the dentist in private that the patient exhibits what she feels could be a moderately advanced stage of periodontal disease. The probing revealed numerous six-millimeter pockets and the tissue was inflamed and enlarged. The dentist responded, "Don't worry; it has been that way for a long time, and I think we can maintain her with cleaning periodically." The dentist tells this to the patient and then moves on to another patient.

The hygienist then tells the patient that she is not comfortable doing only a scaling, so maybe the patient should reschedule at another time with the other hygienist in the office. When the patient heard this, she asked what the hygienist would do if she were in this position. The hygienist replied, "I would see a periodontist."

QUESTIONS

1 Does this case involve legal issues?
2 What are the principles involved in this case?
3 Using the ethical decision-making model, analyze this case.

CASE 2

To Sell or Not To Sell

THOMAS K. HASEGAWA
Baylor College of Dentistry
CARLA LOIACONO
Institute of Medical Education

Dr. Chris Hunt has been in private practice for 10 years in a suburb of a large metropolitan city. Dr. Hunt graduated from an Advanced Education in General Dentistry Program (AEGD) and was an associate in a large general practice for 3 years before buying a building and opening a solo practice. All phases of general dentistry are performed in his practice, but the focus is moving toward adult esthetic dentistry. Ms. Lisa Meyer is a dental hygienist who has been in Dr. Hunt's practice full time for 3 years and enjoys a great relationship with her patients and an active schedule. Ms. Meyer has been a full-time practitioner for 6 years, and this is the second office in which she has worked. Her greatest professional rewards are the trust that has developed between her and her patients and the improvement she has seen in their oral health.

Dr. Hunt recently completed a continuing education series on esthetic dentistry and hired a practice management company to review the office. The course director and the management team both stressed the importance of using the hygienist to "sell dentistry" to patients. The course and the management team both identified certain phrases and inferences hygienists should use to help the patient make the "right" choice.

Dr. Hunt approaches Ms. Meyer and explains her new role to her. Ms. Meyer is uncomfortable with this change in her job duties because she believes she would be using her professional position to possibly unduly influence patients toward making certain treatment choices. "Am I taking advantage of the trust that I worked hard to establish with our patients?" she asks. "No," Dr. Hunt replies. "Actually, you are educating our patients about the benefits of the highest quality care. In fact, to make this arrangement more attractive I am including an incentive plan with cash bonuses for every service that you sell." This statement concerns Ms. Meyer because she believes that these incentives may eventually place her own economic self-interest in conflict with the patient's best interest.

QUESTIONS

1 What aspects of informed consent are important to this case?
2 What are your obligations to your patient as a dental hygienist?
3 What does the ADHA Code say about this type of situation?
4 Relate adult esthetic dentistry to current standards of care.
5 According to the ethical decision-making model, what action should Ms. Meyer take?

CASE 3

Trevor and the Technology

PATRICIA J. NUNN
Utah College of Dental Hygiene

Trevor Wilson, RDH, BSDH. How great that sounded, especially as Trevor began his new job—a job that at least two of his classmates wanted as badly as he did. Dr. Reeves seemed to have the same philosophy as Trevor, she paid exceptionally well, and the office is state of the art.

On his first day Trevor was thrilled to have made it through the first two patients without going over the allotted appointment times, and he did everything according to what he had learned about standard of care. The third patient of the day was 21-year-old Kaleigh Ballantine. Dr. Reeves requested that Trevor use the electronic caries detector because Ms. Ballantine was new to the practice and had not had a thorough hard tissue assessment. Trevor even gloated a little since he was quite familiar with the device. Trevor charted only one reading that strongly indicated a carious lesion, but he also noted several borderline readings on the chart because he knew Dr. Reeves was a perfectionist and would want to know all possible trouble areas as she was evaluating potential lesions visually and tactilely during the examination.

Dr. Reeves sat down for the examination, chatted with Ms. Ballantine, and scanned the dentition with a mouth mirror. She looked at the charting of the potentially carious lesions and said, "Kaleigh, you have a significant number of problems." It looks like you are going to need fillings. We will want to do white ones, of course, because of all the bad news about our trusty silver fillings. The ballpark cost will be around $2100. "Trevor, make sure Kaleigh gets on my schedule so that we can get all these carious lesions taken care of before she gets into trouble. Have the girls up front schedule quadrant by quadrant." Trevor sat dumbfounded.

QUESTIONS

1 What action, if any, should Trevor immediately take?
2 What ethical standards may have been violated?
3 What legal principles may be at risk?
4 Looking at the events through Dr. Reeves' eyes, how might she view the situation?
5 Trevor was really excited about this new job for a number of reasons. Could he have avoided being placed in this situation?
6 How can Trevor avoid putting his job in jeopardy as he resolves this dilemma?
7 According to the ethical decision-making model, what action should Trevor take, if any, after the patient is gone?

CASE 4

A Great Boss

PAMELA ZARKOWSKI
University of Detroit Mercy

Lesa Lawrence thoroughly enjoyed practicing as a dental hygienist. Working in a practice that provided quality patient care was important to her. She also enjoyed being part of a good "team" and the camaraderie of the dental office. Employees sometimes ate lunch in the office and on occasion went out to lunch as a group.

Dr. Frank Harris, Lesa's boss, usually went out to lunch by himself or to meet another dentist. After lunch, Lesa noticed that Dr. Harris frequently smelled like alcohol. She picked up on the same smell in the morning but also noticed he always used mouthrinse before examining a patient. She wanted to believe that she smelled the mouthrinse but was suspicious that it was the smell of alcohol. Lesa mentioned her concern to her fellow employees. They acknowledged that Dr. Harris had a history of alcoholism, seemed to be managing it through Alcoholics Anonymous, but recently had started drinking again. His dental assistant, Corey, assured Lesa that when he appeared unsteady or tentative, she helped out to ensure patient care went smoothly.

Lesa suggested to the office manager that she wanted to help Dr. Harris by reporting him to the state dental society, which had a program to assistant dentists with a substance abuse problem. The office manager, Debbie, became protective of Dr. Harris. She indicated all the staff was receiving generous salaries and if Dr. Harris had to stop practicing to participate in a recovery program, the staff could lose their jobs and their incomes. She reminded Lesa that this had been an ongoing problem and that *all* the staff worked together to "help" Dr. Harris when he was in a compromised state. Debbie reminded Lesa they were a "team" and needed to work together.

QUESTIONS

1 What are the ethical and potential legal issues involved?
2 Does your state practice act address "compromised" practitioners or practitioners with substance abuse problems?
3 Does the ADHA or ADA Code of Ethics specifically address the issues in this case?
4 Using the ethical decision-making model, analyze this case.

CASE 5

Patients with Special Needs

MICHELLE CARR
The Ohio State University

Nancy has been working for the past year as a dental hygienist in a very busy ambulatory health care facility that treats persons who have intellectual and developmental disabilities. The majority of patients treated at this facility are covered under government assistance plans. When procedures are not covered by the insurance plan, the facility writes off the charge for the services. After working in this setting, Nancy found that the patients' oral hygiene generally was poor regardless of whether they were capable of oral hygiene procedures or if they depended on caregivers to brush their teeth. In spite of having dedicated numerous hours training caregivers and providing oral hygiene instruction to the patients, Nancy has met with little success.

Nancy recently implemented a program in which patients who are periodontally involved or had poor oral hygiene were instructed to return for 3-month visits instead of the usual 6-month visits. This approach worked in her previous private practice and had positive results. However, in this new facility, she is not seeing any improvement and questions the value, time, and cost to treat these patients when the facility is not being compensated and no real benefit to the patient is seen. Many patients wait months to get a dental hygiene appointment, and eliminating unresponsive patients on a 3-month visit schedule would allow more appointments for those who are waiting. Nancy is frustrated and wonders how to balance dental needs and economics with these special people.

QUESTIONS

1 What ethical principles is Nancy weighing in this case?
2 What legal principles may be at risk?
3 Using the ethical decision-making model, determine what action Nancy should take.

CASE 6

Standard Precautions

DONNA WITTMAYER
Clark College

A dental hygiene student was assigned to an extramural site where dental care was provided to underserved populations. That morning, as she was reviewing the charts of the patients she would be treating that day, she noted one of the patients was HIV positive and had a history of hepatitis C. The student understood the principles of and always practiced standard precaution procedures; thus she was not concerned about treating the patient. Before this patient's appointment time the dental assistant at the site approached the dental hygiene student and directed her to their supply of disposable lab coats. The assistant stated "You should wear one of these when treating this patient so your cloth lab coat will be not become contaminated." She also instructed the student to place contaminated instruments in a special container of disinfecting solution after she had completed treatment on the patient. After the contaminated instruments had soaked for 30 minutes, they would be processed through the ultrasonic bath and then run through the Chemiclave twice to guarantee the instruments were completely sterilized.

QUESTIONS

1 Should the student follow the recommended procedures at the extramural site, or should she follow the accepted standard procedures? What are the alternatives for the student?
2 Determine the relevant information in this case.
3 Who are the stakeholders affected in this situation?
4 Determine the ethical, legal, or social issues apparent in this situation.
5 Determine the consequences for all stakeholders, both pro and con, most likely to occur for each alternative.
6 Using the ethical decision-making model, analyze this case.

CASE 7

Warming Up

GARY CHIODO
Oregon Health & Science University

A recently graduated dental hygienist has taken a position in a group practice periodontal office. The professional staff in this office includes four periodontists and six dental hygienists. Although she has been on the job only 3 months, the dental hygienist is enjoying the advanced level of practice involved in caring for the patients. Patients referred to this specialty practice are in need of various types of periodontal therapy, and the periodontists maximize the dental hygienists' talents in performing nonsurgical interventions. This dental hygienist has observed the degree of care and thoroughness demonstrated by the periodontists and other hygienists, and she respects their abilities and level of professionalism.

For the past few weeks, however, she has been bothered by one of the periodontists who seems to frequently make inappropriate comments about her appearance, tease her about private body parts, tell her sexually oriented jokes, and constantly ask her to go out on a date with him. Lately this doctor has begun giving her neck and shoulder massages in the employee break room if he finds her there alone. She has asked him to stop because these actions make her uncomfortable and has politely explained that she is not interested in dating him. These protests have not deterred the amorous advances of this dentist, who is recently divorced and vocal about being "in the marketplace."

Today, while the dental hygienist is in her operatory sharpening instruments, the dentist comes in and begins rubbing her neck and shoulders. She rises from her chair and asks him to please stop and to confine his future interactions with her to professional issues. The dentist becomes upset at this rejection and says "You know, I control a significant part of your salary. I don't see why you are always brushing me aside. You'd be lucky to have someone like me. Maybe you should think more about your future here and warm up a little."

QUESTIONS

1 What ethical issues arise from this scenario, and who may be affected by them (e.g., the immediate dental hygienist, the other dental hygienists, the other dentists, patients)?
2 Should the dental hygienist consider any legal issues?
3 How might the dental hygienist deal with this situation while not creating animosity between herself and others in the office?
4 Should she be concerned about creating animosity?
5 How would the ethical and legal issues and the approach change if the person making the amorous advances was another dental hygienist (female) or a female dentist rather than the male dentist?

CASE 8

Patient Confession

DEBRA L. GERGER
West Coast University

A 35-year-old woman comes to your office as a regular 6-month recall patient. She has been a patient in the practice since it opened 7 years ago and is always faithful in coming to her appointments. In general, she is in good health. The dentist completed one bridge a few years ago and her probing depths usually are generalized 3 to 4 mm with light supragingival and subgingival calculus localized to the lower anterior teeth. Some marginal gingival inflammation is present from poor brushing technique.

This patient has been seen by the same dentist for years. The practice is building, and now with four hygienists employed patients often are scheduled with the first available hygienist. This patient has been seen by a different hygienist and then returns to the hygienist who normally sees her each recall. After the medical history review, the hygienist proceeds to do a full mouth probing and discovers that today's readings are significantly lower than the last visit and continues by complimenting the patient on her great improvements.

The patient then reveals that the last hygienist told her that her pockets were so bad that if she did not brush and floss better she would lose all her teeth. She was also told that her cleaning needed to be done every four months to help control the "mess she was in." The patient said she was taking this information in even though it was delivered in a demeaning manner by the other hygienist while she was being "tortured by the scaling procedure." She was in pain during the visit and for three days afterward. The patient also said her 16-year-old daughter had a cleaning by the same person and was in tears from the pain when she came home. When the daughter's chart was pulled, it said "good oral hygiene and light plaque." This is not the first time you have heard this kind of information about this dental hygienist.

QUESTIONS

1 How would you handle this situation?
2 Would you recommend to the patient that she call the dental board?
3 Would you tell the patient that you have heard these kinds of comments before?
4 Would you say something to the dentist?
5 Would you talk with the other dental hygienist?

CASE 9

The Challenge of the Public as a Patient

KATHRYN ANN ATCHISON
University of California at Los Angeles

Betsy Haskell, President of City West Dental Hygienists' Association, put down the telephone and thought about this latest request. The city was planning a strong push for an extensive taxpayer-supported public health program for children. The program was designed to contain a school-based fluoride rinse program and sealant placement using dental hygienists as the driving force and community lay leaders as the personnel for implementing the program.

On the telephone was Dr. Martin Phelps, a well-known local dentist and delegate to the state dental association. He mentioned the association's concern that the frequency of fluorosis in school-age children was growing and that a program, particularly one directed by allied and lay personnel, was extremely risky because of the risk of causing additional fluorosis. Furthermore, he argued, with the recent advances in oral health, few children really experienced serious dental caries. Those who experienced caries were concentrated in a small percentage of poorly educated individuals who failed to maintain good oral health. Therefore whether taxpayer dollars should be used to help children who refused to accept responsibility for maintaining good oral health was questionable.

Betsy listened politely and suggested she might bring the association's concerns to her executive board and get back to him whether they would withdraw their support of the program.

QUESTIONS

1   How are priorities evaluated when considering public health programs? Are fluorosis and caries of equal imperative when weighing the risks and benefits for disadvantaged children? What principles and values are involved?

2   Do oral health professionals have different responsibilities to highly educated versus poorly educated adults? Are there differences in responsibility for poorly educated children? What about people who, because of ignorance, fail to maintain their oral health?

3   Should all dental professionals be obligated or encouraged to promote the same "agenda" for a public health program? On what should the dental professional's "agenda" be based?

4   What would you do if you were Betsy?

CASE 10

Changing the Protocol

MICHELLE M. SINGLEY
Lewis and Clark Community College

You have been employed by Dr. Susan Schneider as a full-time dental hygienist for more than 5 years. You accepted the position because of her sincere devotion to patients' needs and the opportunity she offered to be involved in all phases of patient treatment. At the interview, she stated that she even wanted you to write a "draft" treatment plan based on your findings during the dental hygiene appointment so that she could simply agree or revise the plan as needed when she examined the patient at the end of the hygiene appointment. For 5 years this treatment plan arrangement has worked smoothly, and she even compliments you in front of patients on your excellent skills and dental hygiene diagnostic abilities.

Dr. Schneider is experiencing some personal and professional financial difficulties because of her divorce 6 months ago. She has openly discussed this with all staff, and some office solutions for "cutting back" have been recommended at staff meetings and accepted for implementation.

You begin to see some changes in her methods for treatment planning. Patients who would historically have been treatment planned for a two-surface amalgam are now being treatment planned for crowns. This is not the protocol she followed for the first 5 years you worked with her. You would never disagree with her diagnosis and treatment decisions in the presence of a patient, but you are concerned that patients are being overly treatment planned.

QUESTIONS

1 What would you do in this situation?
2 Does this case have any legal considerations?
3 Using the ethical decision-making model, analyze this case.

CASE 11

The Other Hygienist

MARCIA A. GLADWIN AND CHRISTINA B. DEBIASE
West Virginia University

Sue is a dental hygienist who had 2 years of working experience when she took a new job in an office with another hygienist. This hygienist has been with the practice for 11 years and relies on this job to meet her financial obligations. Sue and this hygienist developed a friendship and often go to lunch together.

Sue has noticed that many patients have subgingival calculus after the other hygienist cleaned their teeth only 3 or 4 months before. One patient even commented to Sue that the other hygienist did not "clean as deep" as she did. When Sue had the opportunity to watch the other hygienist, she found that she exclusively uses an anterior sickle instrument and only scales supragingivally. Sue's immediate reaction was to inform her dentist employer. He replied, "Can you remove it?" Sue answered, "of course I can." The dentist responded, "then remove it." Sue feels the need to do something but has no immediate solution.

QUESTIONS

1 What would you do if you were Sue and why?
2 What ethical principles are involved in this situation?
3 Does Sue have an obligation to the other hygienist?
4 Does the dentist employer have any ethical or legal responsibility?
5 Using the ethical decision-making model, analyze this case.

CASE 12

The Mid-Level Practitioner

ANNE HIGH
Rochester Community and Technical College

Molly is a dental hygienist employed as an oral health practitioner in a state that licenses the mid-level practitioner to provide an expanded scope of practice in underserved areas of the state. The oral health practitioner practices under the general supervision of a licensed dentist in the state and is able to perform simple extractions, restore teeth, perform some pulp therapies, and write prescriptions for a limited range of drugs. A formal collaborative agreement between the dentist and oral health practitioner must be on record with the state board of dentistry. The dentist must be involved in the diagnosis and treatment planning for all patients.

Under normal circumstances, Molly uses the rural dental clinic teledentistry capabilities and communicated with the dentist by live video conference. This arrangement allows the dentist to assist in diagnosis and treatment planning for patients with restorative or surgical needs. Most of the patients Molly treats are young children with dental decay, and a variety of procedures often are required while treating the teeth. The treatment plans often include antibiotic regimens, pulp therapy, stainless steel crowns, restorations, and extraction of primary teeth.

On this particular Thursday, Molly was practicing in the rural clinic and received an emergency phone call from the mother of a patient of record. The patient had not completed his treatment plan last summer and was now in acute pain. Although the dentist had helped plan the treatment for the patient 9 months ago, the tooth indicated for a restoration now presented with an infected pulp. Molly often had treated cases similar to this one and knew what the dentist would probably recommend, but he was out of town and unable to be reached for consultation. Because Molly did not want the child to lose the tooth, she went ahead and treated the patient without consulting the dentist.

QUESTIONS

1 What are the ethical issues to consider in this case?
2 Who might be affected by them (e.g., Molly, the dentist she collaborates with, other oral health practitioners, other dentists, patients)?
3 Should Molly consider any legal issues?
4 How could Molly deal with the situation while considering the legal and ethical issues?
5 Using the ethical decision-making model, analyze this case.

CASE 13

Summer Employment

STEPHANIE BOSSENBERGER JAMES
Weber State University

Mary Ann Fisher has been a dental assistant at Dr. Martan's office for the past 5 years. She functions as a chairside dental assistant, exposing radiographs as directed and acting as the infection control officer for the dental office. During this time Mary Ann has been pursuing her education to become a dental hygienist and recently completed her first year of the program. She has been an above-average student both academically and clinically. However, she has stated that she does not understand why becoming a dental hygienist takes so long. Several times during clinic, Mary Ann has been cited by faculty for taking short cuts and avoiding evaluations. Since she was counseled on this behavior she has been more careful with following protocol. Her clinical performance is at an acceptable level for a student completing the first year of instruction.

School ended in mid-May and Mary Ann was able to resume her employment full time in Dr. Martan's office. Dr. Martan is proud of Mary Ann and often boasts to patients of her accomplishments and that she will be a hygienist very soon. Mary Ann continued with the work she had done in the office for a year, polishing the patient's teeth before the dentist's examination. Now that she has become more adept at instrumentation, she has probed and scaled the teeth of several patients when she has considered it necessary.

Susan, the part-time hygienist in the office, knew that Mary Ann was stretching her dental assisting duties, and after careful consideration decided it was time to have a meeting to talk about what was going on in the office. At the meeting Susan gave out copies of the Dental Practice Act, and everyone understood the reason for the clarification of duties. The dentist thanked Susan and said he thought it was "very informative and interesting." For 6 weeks Mary Ann was careful to only provide services that were listed in the Dental Practice Act. Then she began scaling and probing teeth again.

Susan was disappointed in the dentist and the dental assistant because she thought they would adhere to the legal scope of practice after their meeting. Although Susan was a bit anxious about being fired, she was quite sure that Dr. Martan would understand her concerns for the patients in his practice and not want them to receive substandard care. The more she thought about the situation, the angrier she became. She realized that she is required to report to the board of dental practice any infraction of the state dental practice act.

QUESTIONS

1 Should Susan call the dental hygiene program faculty?
2 Should she tell Dr. Martan that she is going to report this infraction before she does?
3 How serious is the legal infraction?
4 Using the ethical decision-making model, analyze this case.

CASE 14

Program Funds

JOHN ODOM
The Ohio State University

Leslie Tompkins, a hygienist with a masters degree in public health, moved to Ohio from West Virginia 2 years ago. While searching for a position in public health she worked as a hygienist for several practitioners. Six months ago she finally found the opportunity she desired, quit private practice, and was employed by the Ohio Department of Health through funds provided by a recently funded federal special projects grant. Although her job requires her to travel to several counties in the Western part of the state to fulfill her responsibilities, she enjoys her job and sees it as the "stepping stone" needed to move her career forward.

Recently, however, Leslie discovered what she thinks may be illegal management of grant funds by Richard Matheur, regional director and administrator of the special projects grant. Richard is a well-respected member of the community who has ties to the local politicians who were responsible for hiring him. She believes that money is being paid for people who are not eligible to receive it and that these program funds are being redirected to other local projects instead of the special projects and population approved under the grant. After discussing her concerns with Dr. Wiseman, her superior and state director of dental health, she is uncertain about what should be done. Dr. Wiseman told her to use her judgment and "do what you think is right."

QUESTIONS

1 How professional and ethical is the behavior of Dr. Wiseman?
2 What are the consequences if Leslie brings an action (of any sort) against Richard Matheur?
3 What are the consequences if Leslie does nothing?
4 What ethical principles should guide Leslie's decision making?
5 What are the costs of behaving ethically?
6 What are the rewards for ethical behavior?
7 How much should one be asked to sacrifice in the name of ethical and professional behavior?

CASE 15

The Code

PHYLLIS L. BEEMSTERBOER
Oregon Health & Science University

Brad is in his first year of dental school at a well-respected university on the East Coast. He is the first person in his family to go to a professional school and the pride and joy of his large community, all of which are recent immigrants to the United States. His church as well as his extended family are supporting him while he is getting his education. The dental school curriculum is very demanding, and as the first round of examinations approaches Brad is getting more and more concerned that he will not perform well. Other students in his class are talking about "review packets"—old tests from previous years passed down from upper classmates. Several of the old tests in the review packet are the exact examinations one professor gives year after year; he never changes any questions. Using these tests to prepare for the final examinations would save a great deal of time and allow Brad to concentrate on his laboratory courses.

The honor code that Brad signed when he started at the university did not say anything about not using old tests.

QUESTIONS

1 If Brad uses the review packets, is it academic honesty or dishonesty? Why?
2 Do the dental school and its professors have a responsibility in this situation?
3 Are certain types of courses in dental hygiene school more important than others?
4 If you were Brad, what would you do?

CASE 16

My Brother

KATHLEEN H. ALVAREZ
Cypress College

A 35-year-old woman comes to your office for a routine prophylaxis. She has been a patient in the practice for the last 5 years. Upon reviewing and updating the medical history, the patient volunteers that she has recently learned she is HIV positive. She is direct about it and almost flippantly states, "I guess I was a bit wild in my younger days." You note the change to the medical history along with the current medications she is taking and have her fill out a new medical history as well. The appointment proceeds normally, with you discussing the possible oral manifestations of HIV. You provide oral hygiene instructions and advice for caring for her mouth.

Three months later, you are attending a family social function. In walks your brother and your patient. Your brother introduces her as his new girlfriend and indeed seems quite fond of her. When she is introduced to you, she does not appear concerned that you are aware of her HIV status. As the function goes on, you become increasingly uncomfortable with her behavior and intimacy with your brother.

QUESTIONS

1 Do you tell your brother about her HIV status, breaching the patient/ practitioner confidentiality?
2 Can you justify breaching this confidentiality because it is your brother?

3 Do you discuss your concerns with the patient and tell her you will speak with your brother if she does not?

4 How would this affect the professional aspect of the practice you work in?

5 Would you discuss this dilemma with your employer?

6 What are the legal ramifications if you do disclose confidential information to your brother? From the patient? From the employer dentist?

7 What are the personal consequences you will face if you do or do not disclose information?

CASE 17

The Maxillary Bridge

MARY TURNER
Sacramento City College

Dr. Agar, my dentist employer, has the Timothy family—father, mother, and two young daughters—as patients. They are a struggling lower middle class family trying to pay for their daughters' college education. The family has recently received an employee family health policy with dental coverage. Before receiving this coverage, paying for dental care was always a large problem. Unfortunately, Mr. Timothy lost his job 2 weeks ago and is now looking for other employment.

At this time Mr. Timothy is in the middle of several appointments for periodontal debridement before the placement of a new maxillary anterior bridge. Mr. Timothy has asked Dr. Agar to post-date an insurance claim form so that his treatment is covered by the dental plan. Because Dr. Agar would like to help his patient, he has asked me to alter the dates of the dental hygiene services that I will be providing to Mr. Timothy so they also can be included on the claim form.

Mr. Timothy needs the treatment, especially because he is looking for new employment. I know the family well because one of the daughters used to baby-sit for my daughter; they need whatever benefits the insurance will pay.

QUESTIONS

1 Should I comply with Dr. Agar's wishes? After all, he is my boss.

2 What are the ethical and legal issues here?

3 What are the principles involved in this situation?

CASE 18

The Shy Patient

CHERYL A. CAMERON
University of Washington

A new pediatric patient presented for a dental prophylaxis with the dental hygienist. She was an 8-year-old, shy, reserved child who was cute and well mannered. The dental hygienist took an immediate liking to this patient. She had generally good personal and oral health. However, her maxillary central incisors were fractured. When asked about how these teeth were fractured she reported having fallen off her bike. Unfortunately, she was not wearing a helmet. At her recall appointment 6 months later, the dental hygienist noticed that although her incisors were restored, she had bruising around both eyes. When asked about the bruising she reported having fallen down the stairs at home. Her mother was present in the room and held her hand but offered no further explanation. A review of the patient record revealed that this patient sought care by three different general dentists in the same city before transferring her care to the current office.

QUESTIONS

1 Should the dental hygienist suspect child abuse?
2 What professional obligations does the dental hygienist have to the patient?
3 How should the dental hygienist document his or her observations?
4 How should the dental hygienist proceed?

CASE 19

Conflicting Guidelines

KIM L. HALULA
Marquette University

Melissa Morgan is a May graduate of a local community college dental hygiene program. Although her family dentist, Dr. Steven Cain, has been practicing for more than 25 years, he had never employed a dental hygienist before. Melissa was thrilled when Dr. Cain approached her and offered her a job as his first dental hygienist.

Upon graduation, Dr. Cain wanted Melissa to start working immediately. Although Melissa had successfully completed her written and clinical boards and graduated from an accredited dental hygiene program, Melissa informed Dr. Cain that she could not begin working as a dental hygienist until her state dental hygiene license had been issued. Although disappointed, Dr. Cain agreed to wait.

Two weeks after starting her job, Melissa noticed that a number of the health histories for her upcoming patients for the week indicated that the patients needed to be premedicated. In reviewing their health histories, Melissa noted that in each instance the patient was being premedicated because of mitral valve prolapse or rheumatic heart disease.

Melissa remembered learning in her classes that the American Heart Association, with input from the American Dental Association, had released new guidelines for antibiotic premedication in April 2007. The new guidelines state that "antibiotic premedication was no longer indicated for dental patients with mitral valve prolapse; rheumatic heart disease; bicuspid valve disease; calcified aortic stenosis; or congenital heart conditions, such as ventricular septal defects, atrial septal defects, and hypertrophic cardiomyopathy."

Thinking that Dr. Cain might not be aware of this new protocol, Melissa approached him about the new guidelines. Dr. Cain's response shocked Melissa. Not only did he tell her that he had no intention of changing his premedication policy, he also instructed her not to mention these new standards to any of his patients currently receiving premedication.

Dr. Cain also informed Melissa that he believed she was too idealistic. He was reconsidering whether he really needed a dental hygienist because he had practiced for more than 25 years without one and had no problems and now he believed his practices and ethics were being questioned.

QUESTIONS

1 What are the issues here?
2 Using the ethical decision-making model, analyze this case.

CASE 20

Integrity Protocol

DONNA LESSER
Riverside Community College

While teaching the general pathology course, Ms. Sally Samson believed she detected a student attempting to cheat on a quiz. The student appeared to have written information on her leg. Ms. Samson believed she could not confirm this and decided to watch the student more closely before making an allegation that could not be substantiated. Over the next 2 weeks Ms. Samson gave two more quizzes in her pathology course. She was almost certain that the student in question had terms written on the palms of her hands and that she manipulated her hands in a way to view the information during the quizzes.

Ms. Samson took her suspicions to the director of the program. The program director told her that no other faculty member had presented concerns about this student but that she had found pathology words written on the table in the classroom where the pathology course was held. To complicate matters, the program director told Ms. Samson that the student's father was a senior faculty member at the institution who was on the faculty council and heavily involved in the teachers' union. With this information, they decided that Ms. Samson would try to eliminate the student's questionable behavior by implementing additional protocols to make cheating "too much work." One new protocol was to have each student apply an alcohol spray to their hands before taking a quiz or examination.

Approximately 4 weeks later, Ms. Samson was giving a mid-term examination and had the students line up to use the alcohol spray. When the student in question turned her hands over, Ms. Samson saw terms written on the palms of her hands. She tapped the student on the shoulder and told her to report to the director's office. On the way out of the room, the student vigorously wiped her palms on her jeans to remove the writing. By the time the student arrived in the director's office she had vague outlines of ink on her hands.

QUESTIONS

1 How should the program director handle this situation?
2 Did Ms. Samson deal with this problem well?
3 Should all allegations of cheating be reviewed by an honor council?
4 What role should students in the class play in this dilemma?

CASE 21

Such a Deal

PHYLLIS MARTINA
Hu-Friedy Manufacturing Company, Inc.

Camille is a second-year dental hygiene student who has accepted the responsibility for organizing the instrument orders for her class. She is the class president and is well respected by her classmates and faculty members. Camille is aware that companies offer a greatly reduced price for student purchases; in fact, the price reduction is significant—often 60% less than manufacturers' suggested retail price.

One of the clinical faculty members has asked Camille to place an order at the student price for her use in her private practice. Knowing that the student price is offered for students only, what should she do?

QUESTIONS

1 How should she handle this situation?
2 Is this a legal problem?
3 Using the ethical decision-making model, analyze this case.

CASE 22

The Diagnosis Hygienist

GAIL AAMODT
Pacific University

Marilyn has been employed in the same dental office for the past 8 years and loves the people she works with. A new dentist has recently joined the dental team and is scheduled on the same days as Marilyn. The new dentist is from a foreign country and appears to not have a very high opinion of women, being somewhat rude to the staff, especially when the owner of the practice is not in the office.

After several weeks it becomes clear that his dentistry is not of the same high quality as the other dentists in the practice. Marilyn is removing more overhangs than ever before and has noticed several open margins. In addition, he is diagnosing more crowns than any other dentist in the practice and recently placed a crown on a periodontally involved tooth.

Marilyn has tried discussing her concerns with him and was told that he is the dentist and she does not know what she is talking about. He said that Marilyn is speaking outside her knowledge and skill level and reminded her that dental hygienists cannot diagnose dental disease. He even told her that she would regret it if she continued with these "wild accusations" of his work.

QUESTIONS

1 Is this an ethical or legal situation?
2 Using the ethical decision-making model, analyze this case.

CASE 23

Fitting In

PAMELA OVERMAN
University of Missouri–Kansas City

Sarah is happy to have a job as a dental hygienist for Dr. Stanley Dard. Sarah is a newly divorced mother of two teenagers and must stay in this geographic area as a part of the divorce settlement. Dr. Dard is a member of the state dental board who highly values the periodontal aspect of care. He serves as a state clinical examiner, and he checks patients meticulously to make sure everyone receives the best care. Recently, however, Sarah has seen a side of Dr. Dard that has her concerned. She walked by his operatory as he was presenting a proposed treatment plan to a new patient. The patient was a devout Muslim woman wearing traditional loose-fitting dress and a scarf covering her hair. When discussing the fees with the patient, Dr. Dard quoted fees that were *considerably* higher than those he typically presents. Sarah assumed she misheard until it happened again—to a male Hispanic patient with limited English language skills. Sarah waits for an opportune moment and asks Dr. Dard about how he sets fees for services when presenting treatment plans. He says he sets fees based on difficulty of the treatment and seems disinclined to go into much more depth.

Today Sarah sees a treatment plan presentation on Dr. Dard's schedule. When she walks by the treatment room, the door is closed. After the final patient of the day, Dr. Dard asks Sarah to stop by his office for a discussion about her performance in his office. He is not sure Sarah fits in. Sarah is panicked and not sure what to do next.

QUESTIONS

1 What action, if any, should Sarah take immediately?
2 What ethical standards might have been violated?
3 What legal principles may be at risk?
4 How might Dr. Dard view this situation?

5 Could Sarah have avoided being placed in this situation?

6 Using the ethical decision-making model, what action should Sarah take, if any?

CASE 24

New Skills

ANN LOUISE MCCANN
Baylor College of Dentistry

The ability to treat children was the reason that Harper Mallone, RDH, went to dental hygiene school. She loved working at the office of Dr. Marvin Stallsworth because it was a family practice, and she got the opportunity to treat many children. She hoped to have her own children someday; caring for them was her special love and she was good at it.

Dr. Stallsworth believed in saving as much tooth structure as possible and often did sealants on teeth with small occlusal carious lesions. This procedure (called an enameloplasty) involved excavating only the carious enamel tissue with a small bur and then placing a sealant in the area. Harper would identify the carious lesions during her oral examination at patient recall appointments. When Dr. Stallsworth came into the dental hygiene operatory for his examination of the patient, he would prepare the tooth and then have Harper place the sealant.

One morning, Dr. Stallsworth requested that Harper learn how to do an enameloplasty so that she could perform the entire sealant procedure herself. He said it was quite easy to do and it would free him up to spend more time with his restorative patients. This would be a win-win situation for both the office and the patient by decreasing the length of the dental hygiene appointment. When the next patient arrived who needed a sealant, Dr. Stallsworth showed Harper how to do the enameloplasty and had her use a high-speed handpiece to remove the carious enamel. Harper found the procedure fairly easy and was looking forward to doing the procedure on future patients.

She enthusiastically described her new skill to a fellow dental hygienist at the monthly dental hygiene society meeting. Her friend expressed surprise that she was placing sealant restorations and told her she should not be restoring teeth. Harper did not know what to do. Her employer wanted her to do the procedure independently, and she liked having more responsibility at the office.

QUESTION

1 Using the ethical decision-making model, analyze this case.

CASE 25

Penny Wise, Pound Foolish

PHYLLIS L. BEEMSTERBOER, CATHERINE SALVESON, KAREN ADAMS
Oregon Health & Science University

Melissa is a 19-year-old woman who is at 27 weeks' gestation in her first pregnancy who presents for her first prenatal visit at County Health Clinic. She has not seen a health care provider thus far because she has not had coverage; she works at a local pizza restaurant, and her employer does not provide health insurance. The clinic social worker enrolled her in the Oregon Health Plan (a safety net program) and explained that she would have coverage during her pregnancy. Melissa lives with her sister in an apartment and does not have a car of her own. Her sister drives her to work or she takes the bus, so traveling to clinic visits is difficult for her.

The nurse practitioner at the clinic determined that Melissa's pregnancy has been uncomplicated thus far. She had some nausea and vomiting in the first trimester that had resolved, and she had not had any bleeding or contractions. Her history was significant for a previous abnormal Pap smear that she had not followed up and chlamydia that was treated as an outpatient 2 years ago. Melissa smokes a little over a pack of cigarettes per day and denies using alcohol or recreational drugs during the pregnancy. She has begun prenatal vitamins. She is in a monogamous relationship with the father of the baby, who is currently incarcerated for theft. They have been together for 2 years and plan to marry when he is released next year.

Melissa's examination was consistent with 27 weeks' gestation, and the nurse practitioner performed a Pap and cervical cultures. She drew prenatal laboratory values and set Melissa up with an appointment for an ultrasound, although Melissa was not sure she would be able to get time off work for the appointment. She stated that her boss was strict about time away from work, and she was afraid she would lose her job if she missed too much time.

The nurse noticed that Melissa's dentition was very poor and inquired when her last dental examination had been. Melissa could not remember but believed that it was at least several years ago. She admitted to some right-sided jaw pain. The nurse gave her the names of several dentists in the area and encouraged her to schedule an appointment. Melissa wanted to know if dental care would be covered on the Oregon Health Plan because she was afraid of a large dental bill that she could not pay.

The next week Melissa presented by ambulance to the emergency department with premature onset of contractions. The labor and delivery physician obtained the records from the clinic and found that her chlamydia culture was positive and that the clinic had been unable to contact Melissa because her phone had been disconnected. The obstetrician treated Melissa with medication to stop her contractions, gave her antibiotics for the chlamydia infection, and looked for any other infections because infection is a common cause of premature labor. He found an abscessed molar on her right side. The next day Melissa's drug screen returned positive for opiates.

After 2 days in the hospital a reviewer from the Oregon Health Plan indicated to her attending physician that her preterm labor was believed to be arrested enough that Melissa should be discharged. The physician did so, giving her strict instructions to see a dentist within the week to deal with the abscess, explaining to her that her preterm labor might return if she did not do so. He also explained to her that the positive drug screen meant that Child Protective Services would need to be involved after her baby was born. Six days later Melissa returned to the hospital, having delivered her infant at 29 weeks' gestation in the ambulance on the way to the hospital. Her infant was immediately taken to the neonatal intensive care unit (NICU), where it was placed on mechanical ventilation for respiratory distress syndrome. Melissa had not seen a dentist and still had the abscessed tooth. The NICU nurse discussed her baby's expected hospital course with Melissa, telling her as gently as she could that the baby would likely be in the hospital for 5 to 6 weeks and could potentially have long-term mental retardation, blindness, and chronic lung disease. Melissa looked around at the monitors and equipment in the NICU and her tiny baby and wondered how she would be able to pay for it all. She told herself that she would worry about the bills later, and told the nurse "I want everything possible done for my baby."

QUESTION

1 You are a member of the hospital review board who has been assigned to review this situation. Using the ethical decision-making model, analyze this case.

▪ Testlets

Testlet 1

Virginia is a dental hygienist in a busy practice with three dentists, one other hygienist, and six dental assistants. The office also supports an administrative staff of four. Oak Grove Dentistry is a high-volume practice, with 250 to 300 patient visits per week among the clinical practitioners. New patients to the practice are seen first by the dental hygienists, who take the medical history and perform the initial examination, including the current periodontal status and restorative needs.

Although Virginia is impressed by the quality of services that the patients receive, she is distressed by what she believes is a wide disparity between her clinical assessment of restorative need and that of one of the dentists who finds many more carious lesions than she notes. Her observations were confirmed when she discussed the issue with the other hygienist and one of the dentists, both of whom expressed similar concerns.

When Virginia approached Dr. Kane, the owner of the practice, with her concern, she was told clearly that definitive diagnosis of caries and oral disease is within the scope of practice for the dentist, not the dental hygienist. When Virginia added that the other dental hygienist also was concerned, Dr. Kane intimated that she was a "troublemaker" and any further allegations that he was not acting in the best interests of his patients would not be tolerated.

1 This case presents issues that may be
   a unethical.
   b illegal.
   c grounds for malpractice.
   d all the above.
   e none of the above.

2 The main principle involved in this case is
   a autonomy.
   b beneficence.
   c nonmaleficence.
   d justice.
   e veracity.

3 Does Virginia have any responsibility to the patients in this practice?
   a No; she is an employee, not the owner, of the practice.
   b Yes; she must adhere to the ADHA Code of Ethics.

Multiple-choice answers for testlet questions are provided on p. 202.

4 What section of the ADHA Code of Ethics "Standards" applies to this situation?
  a "To ourselves as professionals"
  b "To clients"
  c "To employees and employers"
  d "To the dental hygiene profession"
  e "To the community and society"

Testlet 2

A patient assigned to Sarah Smith in the periodontal practice where she works has a severe case of what she thinks is type IV periodontal disease. The dentist employer initially examined the patient, and because of the amount of calculus present, sent her for scaling and debridement. The patient is elderly, somewhat shy, and keeps saying that she wants Sarah to do "whatever is necessary" so she can keep her teeth. Sarah is concerned that the patient does not fully understand her disease, the scope of treatment, and treatment options.

1 What health care obligation is most important in this case?
  a Confidentiality
  b Informed consent
  c Paternalism
  d Veracity

2 Making sure the patient understands the course of treatment is honoring the ethical principle of
  a autonomy.
  b beneficence.
  c justice.
  d nonmaleficence.
  e veracity.

3 Sarah should be concerned about this situation because the patient is
  a elderly and shy.
  b too trusting.
  c yet to be diagnosed by the dentist.
  d not well informed about her oral health.

4 What section of the ADHA Code of Ethics "Standards" applies to this situation?
  a "To ourselves as professionals"
  b "To clients"

   c "To employees and employers"
   d "To the dental hygiene profession"
   e "To the community and society"

Testlet 3

A new patient, Susan, is a 15-year-old single young woman who is seeing a dental hygienist for dental care for the first time. In this practice radiographs are taken of every new patient as part of the diagnostic data gathering. As a safety precaution before taking radiographs, women of childbearing age are asked whether they could be pregnant. Susan, aware that her mother is in the waiting room, very quietly tells the hygienist that she is pregnant. She also says that her parents are unaware of her condition and begs the hygienist not to tell her mother or the dentist.

1 Which main ethical principles are involved for the dental hygienist in this case?
   a Autonomy and nonmaleficence
   b Beneficence and justice
   c Nonmaleficence and veracity
   d Justice and autonomy
   e All the above

2 At what age would this person become an adult?
   a When she turns 16 years of age
   b When she turns 18 years of age
   c When she pays for her own dental care
   d When the state law says she is an adult

3 Taking radiographs of pregnant women is not recommended because
   a radiation is dangerous for a fetus.
   b radiation may be dangerous for a fetus.
   c pregnancy gingivitis is a risk.
   d of concerns for the health of the mother.

4 The dental hygienist should first
   a try to convince Susan to discuss her pregnancy with her mother.
   b inform the dentist of this dilemma.
   c contact Susan's mother and inform her of the pregnancy.
   d delay dental hygiene treatment.

Testlet 4

Julie is a part-time dental assistant and a graduate of an accredited dental assisting program. She was credentialed by the state to expose radiographs and place pit and fissure sealants as expanded functions. She works in a practice the 2 days of the week that the dental hygienist is not scheduled and generally sees a full client load. Many of her clients were children when she began her employment, but lately she has noticed that many of them are now adults on medical assistance.

The dentist explained to her that he would scale the client's teeth and directed Julie to polish them because that is "as good as the hygienist would be able to do." When Julie checked the medical assistance claim form for these clients, she found that her services were being billed as "adult prophylaxis."

The dentist employer told Julie that the medical assistance reimbursement rates were so poor that he believed these clients were getting more than adequate treatment. He pointed out that he was one of the few dentists in the area who provided any treatment to medical assistance patients and that Julie should be happy to assist in this valuable service.

1 This case presents issues that are
  a unethical.
  b illegal.
  c grounds for malpractice.
  d all the above.
  e none of the above.

2 Which ethical principle is most important in this case?
  a Autonomy
  b Beneficence
  c Nonmaleficence
  d Justice
  e Veracity

3 The clinical function of polishing teeth
  a is a traditional dental assisting duty.
  b is an expanded dental assisting duty.
  c is a function of the dental hygienist.
  d can be delegated by the dentist.
  e depends on state law.

▪ Suggested Activities

The following activities can be used to enhance the study of ethics and law in dental hygiene. These activities can be accomplished individually or in small working groups.

1 Explore the medical and nursing literature on medical ethics or bioethics to see the range of references available.

2 Look at a medical textbook on ethics. Compare the types of issues presented and discussed in those books with those presented and discussed in this text.

3 Scan the newspaper and see how many articles, over a certain period, relate to ethical issues. What principle is most often cited?

4 Search the Internet and list the number of sites that refer to dentistry and ethics.

5 Choose one of the following topics and research the issue as it affects health care and health care delivery:
   ▪ Abortion
   ▪ AIDS/HIV infection
   ▪ Access to care
   ▪ Assisted suicide
   ▪ Blood transfusion
   ▪ Clinical and translational research
   ▪ Emergency care
   ▪ Harvesting reproductive cells
   ▪ Health maintenance organizations
   ▪ Informed consent
   ▪ Integrative medicine
   ▪ Law and life support
   ▪ Paternalism
   ▪ Placebos
   ▪ Transplantation

6 Locate the code of ethics from a health care professional group, such as physical therapists, chiropractors, or medical technologists. Compare that code with the ADHA Code.

7 Locate the code of ethics for another medical organization. Compare it with the ADHA Code and/or the ADA Code.

8 Find the website for the American Society for Dental Ethics and explore what the group does.

9 Research the materials available from the following centers for ethical study:
   ▪ Hastings Center, Garrison, NY
   ▪ Center for Health Care Ethics, St. Louis, MO

- Center for Ethics in Health Care, Portland, OR
- Center for Practical Bioethics (formerly Midwest Bioethics Center) Kansas City, MO
- Ethics Institute of Dartmouth College, Hanover, NH
- Kennedy Institute of Ethics, Washington DC

10 Research and list the ethical issues that can arise in relation to dental research.

11 Retrieve a bibliography on a bioethics topic from the National Reference Center for Bioethics Literature.

12 Establish small study groups to explore different cultures and then compare common beliefs and practices.

13 Discuss ethnocentrism and how it can affect the practice of dental hygiene and dentistry.

14 Establish small groups and research the state dental practice acts from several different regions in the United States.

15 Research a recent dental malpractice case in your state or region and identify the risk management errors that may have led to the legal action.

16 Analyze the risk management practices in the clinical setting in which you are working or plan to work.

17 Research the issues surrounding the professional with drug or alcohol impairment and determine how those issues are handled in your state or region, both ethically and legally.

18 Contact your state dental disciplinary body and inquire about the number and type of complaints it receives and how they are resolved.

19 Access your state government website and find out the rights and responsibilities of employers and employees.

20 Explore some of the following websites:

NAME	LOCATION	WEBSITE
American Association for the Advancement of Science		www.aaas.org
Association for Practical and Professional Ethics	Bloomington, IN	www.indiana.edu/~appe
Bioethics Institute	Johns Hopkins University	www.bioethicsinstitute.org
Bioethics Institute	Loyola University Marymount	www.lmu.edu/PageFactory.aspx?PageID=25764

(Continued)

NAME	LOCATION	WEBSITE
Canadian Centre for Ethics & Corporate Policy	Toronto, Ontario, Canada	www.ethicscentre.ca
Case Studies in Education	Utah Valley State College	www.uvsc.edu/ethics/ curriculum/education
Center for Applied Philosophy and Ethics in the Professions	University of Florida	www.ethics.ufl.edu/index. html
Center for Bioethics and Human Dignity	Trinity International University, Illinois	www.cbhd.net
Center for Ethics	Emory College	www.ethics.emory.edu/ index
Center for Ethics and Leadership in the Health Professions	Regis University	www.ethicsandleadership. org
Center for Ethics and Social Justice	Loyola University Chicago	www.luc.edu/depts/ethics
Center for Ethics Education	Fordham University	www.fordham.edu/ academics/office_of_ research/research_ centers__in/center_for_ ethics_ed/
Center for Ethics in Health Care	Portland, OR	www.ohsu.edu/ethics
Center for Ethics in the Professions	University of Puerto Rico, Mayaguez	www.uprm.edu/etica
Center for Health Care Ethics	Saint Louis University	http://chce.slu.edu/
Center for Health Policy & Ethics	Creighton University Medical Center	http://chpe.creighton.edu
Center for Law, Ethics, & Health	University of Michigan School of Public Health	www.sph.umich.edu/cleh
Center for Practical Bioethics (formerly known as Midwest Bioethics Center)	Kansas City, MO	http://caringcommunity. org
Center for Research Ethics & Bioethics	Uppsala University (Sweden)	www.crb.uu.se

NAME	LOCATION	WEBSITE
Center for the Study of Ethics	Utah Valley State College	www.uvsc.edu/ethics
Center for the Study of Ethics in Society	Western Michigan University	www.wmich.edu/ethics
Centre for Professional Ethics	University of Central Lancashire, United Kingdom	www.uclan.ac.uk/facs/ health/ethics/index.htm
Dartmouth College Ethics Institute	Hanover, NH	www.dartmouth.edu/ ~ethics
Edmond J. Safra Foundation Center for Ethics	Harvard University	www.ethicsharvard.edu
Ethics Resource Center		www.ethics.org
World Dental Federation (FDI)	Ferney-Voltoire, France	www.fdiworldental.org/ home/home.html
Hastings Center	Garrison, New York	www.thehastingscenter.org
Institute for Business and Professional Ethics	DePaul University, Chicago	www.depaul.edu/ethics
The Institute of Catholic Bioethics	Saint Joseph's University	www.sju.edu/bioethics/ index.html
Josephson Institute	Marina del Ray, CA	www.josephsoninstitute. org
The Kenan Institute for Ethics	Duke University	http://kenan.ethics.duke. edu
The Kennedy Institute of Ethics	Georgetown University	http://kennedyinstitute. georgetown.edu http://bioethics. georgetown.edu
Neiswanger Institute for Bioethics and Health Policy	Loyola University Chicago	http://bioethics.lumc.edu
Research Ethics and Academic Integrity	Syracuse University	http://gradschpdprograms. syr.edu/resources/ videos.php
Vanderbilt University Center for Ethics	Vanderbilt University	www.vanderbilt.edu/ CenterforEthics

Answers to Testlet Questions

Testlet 1

1. d
2. c
3. b
4. b

Testlet 2

1. b
2. a
3. d
4. b

Testlet 3

1. a
2. d
3. b
4. a

Testlet 4

1. d
2. e
3. e

APPENDIX A

American Dental Association *Principles of Ethics and Code of Professional Conduct* with Official Advisory Opinions Revised to October 2008

CONTENTS

The Code of Professional Conduct is organized into five sections. Each section falls under the Principle of Ethics that predominately applies to it. Advisory Opinions follow the section of the Code that they interpret.

I. INTRODUCTION

The dental profession holds a special position of trust within society. As a consequence, society affords the profession certain privileges that are not available to members of the public-at-large. In return, the profession makes a commitment to society that its members will adhere to high ethical standards of conduct. These standards are embodied in the *ADA Principles of Ethics and Code of Professional Conduct (ADA Code)*. The *ADA Code* is, in effect, a written expression of the obligations arising from the implied contract between the dental profession and society.

Members of the ADA voluntarily agree to abide by the *ADA Code* as a condition of membership in the Association. They recognize that continued public trust in the dental profession is based on the commitment of individual dentists to high ethical standards of conduct.

The *ADA Code* has three main components: **The Principles of Ethics, the Code of Professional Conduct** and the **Advisory Opinions**.

The **Principles of Ethics** are the aspirational goals of the profession. They provide guidance and offer justification for the *Code of Professional Conduct* and the *Advisory Opinions*. There are five fundamental principles that form the foundation of the *ADA Code:* patient autonomy, nonmaleficence, beneficence, justice and veracity. Principles can overlap each other as well as compete with each other for priority. More than one principle can justify a given element of the *Code of Professional Conduct.* Principles may at times need to be balanced against each other, but, otherwise, they are the profession's firm guideposts.

The **Code of Professional Conduct** is an expression of specific types of conduct that are either required or prohibited. The *Code of Professional Conduct* is a product of the ADA's legislative system. All elements of the *Code of Professional Conduct* result from resolutions that are adopted by the ADA's House of Delegates. The *Code of Professional Conduct* is binding on members of the ADA, and violations may result in disciplinary action.

The **Advisory Opinions** are interpretations that apply the *Code of Professional Conduct* to specific fact situations. They are adopted by the ADA's Council on Ethics, Bylaws and Judicial Affairs to provide guidance to the membership on how the Council might interpret the *Code of Professional Conduct* in a disciplinary proceeding.

The *ADA Code* is an evolving document and by its very nature cannot be a complete articulation of all ethical obligations. The *ADA Code* is the result of an on-going dialogue between the dental profession and society, and as such, is subject to continuous review.

Although ethics and the law are closely related, they are not the same. Ethical obligations may–and often do–exceed legal duties. In resolving any ethical problem not explicitly covered by the *ADA Code*, dentists should consider the ethical principles, the patient's needs and interests, and any applicable laws.

II. PREAMBLE

The American Dental Association calls upon dentists to follow high ethical standards which have the benefit of the patient as their primary goal. In recognition of this goal, the education and training of a dentist has resulted in society affording to the profession the privilege and obligation of self-government. To fulfill this privilege, these high ethical standards should be adopted and practiced throughout the dental school educational process and subsequent professional career.

The Association believes that dentists should possess not only knowledge, skill and technical competence but also those traits of character that foster adherence to ethical principles. Qualities of honesty, compassion, kindness, integrity, fairness and charity are part of the ethical education of a dentist and practice of dentistry and help to define the true professional. As such, each dentist should share in providing advocacy to and care of the underserved. It is urged that the dentist meet this goal, subject to individual cirsumstances.

The ethical dentist strives to do that which is right and good. The *ADA Code* is an instrument to help the dentist in this quest.

III. PRINCIPLES, CODE OF PROFESSIONAL CONDUCT, AND ADVISORY OPINIONS

Section 1 Principle: Patient Autonomy ("self-governance")

The dentist has a duty to respect the patient's rights to self-determination and confidentiality.

> This principle expresses the concept that professionals have a duty to treat the patient according to the patient's desires, within the bounds of accepted treatment, and to protect the patient's confidentiality. Under this principle, the dentist's primary obligations include involving patients in treatment decisions in a meaningful way, with due consideration being given to the patient's needs, desires and abilities, and safeguarding the patient's privacy.

CODE OF PROFESSIONAL CONDUCT

1.A. Patient Involvement

The dentist should inform the patient of the proposed treatment, and any reasonable alternatives, in a manner that allows the patient to become involved in treatment decisions.

1.B. Patient Records

Dentists are obliged to safeguard the confidentiality of patient records. Dentists shall maintain patient records in a manner consistent with the protection of the welfare of the patient. Upon request of a patient or another dental practitioner, dentists shall provide any information in accordance with applicable law that will be beneficial for the future treatment of that patient.

ADVISORY OPINIONS

1.B.1. Furnishing Copies of Records

A dentist has the ethical obligation on request of either the patient or the patient's new dentist to furnish in accordance with applicable law, either gratuitously or for nominal cost, such dental records or copies or summaries of them, including dental X-rays or copies of them, as will be beneficial for the future treatment of that patient. This obligation exists whether or not the patient's account is paid in full.

1.B.2. Confidentiality of Patient Records

The dominant theme in Code Section l.B is the protection of the confidentiality of a patient's records. The statement in this section that relevant information in the records should be released to another dental practitioner assumes that the dentist requesting the information is the patient's present dentist. There may be circumstances where the former dentist has an ethical obligation to inform the present dentist of certain facts. Code Section 1.B assumes that the dentist releasing relevant information is acting in accordance with applicable law. Dentists should be aware, that the laws of the various jurisdictions in the United States are not uniform, and some confidentiality laws appear to prohibit the transfer of pertinent information, such as HIV seropositivity. Absent certain knowledge that the laws of the dentist's jurisdiction permit the forwarding of this information, a dentist should obtain the patient's written permission before forwarding health records which contain information of a sensitive nature, such as HIV seropositivity, chemical dependency or sexual preference. If it is necessary for a treating dentist to consult with another dentist or physician with respect to the patient, and the circumstances do not permit the patient to remain anonymous, the treating dentist should seek the permission of the patient prior to the release of data from the patient's records to the consulting practitioner. If the patient refuses, the treating dentist should then contemplate obtaining legal advice regarding the termination of the dentist/patient relationship.

▓ Section 2 Principle: Nonmaleficence *("do no harm")*

The dentist has a duty to refrain from harming the patient.

> This principle expresses the concept that professionals have a duty to protect the patient from harm. Under this principle, the dentist's

primary obligations include keeping knowledge and skills current, knowing one's own limitations and when to refer to a specialist or other professional, and knowing when and under what circumstances delegation of patient care to auxiliaries is appropriate.

CODE OF PROFESSIONAL CONDUCT

2.A. Education

The privilege of dentists to be accorded professional status rests primarily in the knowledge, skill and experience with which they serve their patients and society. All dentists, therefore, have the obligation of keeping their knowledge and skill current.

2.B. Consultation and Referral

Dentists shall be obliged to seek consultation, if possible, whenever the welfare of patients will be safeguarded or advanced by utilizing those who have special skills, knowledge, and experience. When patients visit or are referred to specialists or consulting dentists for consultation:

1 The specialists or consulting dentists upon completion of their care shall return the patient, unless the patient expressly reveals a different preference, to the referring dentist, or, if none, to the dentist of record for future care.
2 The specialists shall be obliged when there is no referring dentist and upon a completion of their treatment to inform patients when there is a need for further dental care.

ADVISORY OPINION

2.B.1. Second Opinions

A dentist who has a patient referred by a third party[1] for a "second opinion" regarding a diagnosis or treatment plan recommended by the patient's treating dentist should render the requested second opinion in accordance with this *Code of Ethics*. In the interest of the patient being afforded quality care, the dentist rendering the second opinion should not have a vested interest in the ensuing recommendation.

2.C. Use of Auxiliary Personnel

Dentists shall be obliged to protect the health of their patients by only assigning to qualified auxiliaries those duties which can be legally delegated. Dentists shall be further obliged to prescribe and supervise the patient care provided by all auxiliary personnel working under their direction.

2.D. Personal Impairment

It is unethical for a dentist to practice while abusing controlled substances, alcohol or other chemical agents which impair the ability to practice. All dentists have an ethical obligation to urge chemically impaired colleagues to seek treatment. Dentists with first-hand knowledge that a colleague is practicing dentistry when so impaired have an ethical responsibility to report such evidence to the professional assistance committee of a dental society.

ADVISORY OPINION

2.D.1. Ability to Practice

A dentist who contracts any disease or becomes impaired in any way that might endanger patients or dental staff shall, with consultation and advice from a qualified physician or other authority, limit the activities of practice to those areas that do not endanger patients or dental staff. A dentist who has been advised to limit the activities of his or her practice should monitor the aforementioned disease or impairment and make additional limitations to the activities of the dentist's practice, as indicated.

2.E. Postexposure, Bloodborne Pathogens

All dentists, regardless of their bloodborne pathogen status, have an ethical obligation to immediately inform any patient who may have been exposed to blood or other potentially infectious material in the dental office of the need for postexposure evaluation and follow-up and to immediately refer the patient to a qualified health care practitioner who can provide postexposure services. The dentist's ethical obligation in the event of an exposure incident extends to providing information concerning the dentist's own bloodborne pathogen status to the evaluating health care practitioner, if the dentist is the source individual, and to submitting to testing that will assist in the evaluation of the patient. If a staff member or other third person is the source individual, the dentist should encourage that person to cooperate as needed for the patient's evaluation.

2.F. Patient Abandonment

Once a dentist has undertaken a course of treatment, the dentist should not discontinue that treatment without giving the patient adequate notice and the opportunity to obtain the services of another dentist. Care should be taken that the patient's oral health is not jeopardized in the process.

2.G. Personal Relationships with Patients

Dentists should avoid interpersonal relationships that could impair their professional judgment or risk the possibility of exploiting the confidence placed in them by a patient.

▨ Section 3 Principle: Beneficence ("do good")

The dentist has a duty to promote the patient's welfare.

> This principle expresses the concept that professionals have a duty to act for the benefit of others. Under this principle, the dentist's primary obligation is service to the patient and the public-at-large. The most important aspect of this obligation is the competent and timely delivery of dental care within the bounds of clinical circumstances presented by the patient, with due consideration being given to the needs, desires and values of the patient. The same ethical considerations apply whether the dentist engages in fee-for-service, managed care or some other practice arrangement. Dentists may choose to enter into contracts governing the provision of care to a group of patients; however, contract obligations do not excuse dentists from their ethical duty to put the patient's welfare first.

CODE OF PROFESSIONAL CONDUCT

3.A. Community Service

Since dentists have an obligation to use their skills, knowledge and experience for the improvement of the dental health of the public and are encouraged to be leaders in their community, dentists in such service shall conduct themselves in such a manner as to maintain or elevate the esteem of the profession.

3.B. Government of a Profession

Every profession owes society the responsibility to regulate itself. Such regulation is achieved largely through the influence of the professional societies. All dentists, therefore, have the dual obligation of making themselves a part of a professional society and of observing its rules of ethics.

3.C. Research and Development

Dentists have the obligation of making the results and benefits of their investigative efforts available to all when they are useful in safeguarding or promoting the health of the public.

3.D. Patents and Copyrights

Patents and copyrights may be secured by dentists provided that such patents and copyrights shall not be used to restrict research or practice.

3.E. Abuse and Neglect

Dentists shall be obliged to become familiar with the signs of abuse and neglect and to report suspected cases to the proper authorities, consistent with state laws.

ADVISORY OPINION

3.E.1. Reporting Abuse and Neglect

The public and the profession are best served by dentists who are familiar with identifying the signs of abuse and neglect and knowledgeable about the appropriate intervention resources for all populations.

A dentist's ethical obligation to identify and report the signs of abuse and neglect is, at a minimum, to be consistent with a dentist's legal obligation in the jurisdiction where the dentist practices. Dentists, therefore, are ethically obliged to identify and report suspected cases of abuse and neglect to the same extent as they are legally obliged to do so in the jurisdiction where they practice. Dentists have a concurrent ethical obligation to respect an adult patient's right to self-determination and confidentiality and to promote the welfare of all patients. Care should be exercised to respect the wishes of an adult patient who asks that a suspected case of abuse and/or neglect not be reported, where such a report is not mandated by law. With the patient's permission, other possible solutions may be sought.

Dentists should be aware that jurisdictional laws vary in their definitions of abuse and neglect, in their reporting requirements and the extent to which immunity is granted to good faith reporters. The variances may raise potential legal and other risks that should be considered, while keeping in mind the duty to put the welfare of the patient first. Therefore a dentist's ethical obligation to identify and report suspected cases of abuse and neglect can vary from one jurisdiction to another.

Dentists are ethically obligated to keep current their knowledge of both identifying abuse and neglect and reporting it in the jurisdiction(s) where they practice.

Section 4 Principle: Justice *("fairness")*

The dentist has a duty to treat people fairly.

> This principle expresses the concept that professionals have a duty to be fair in their dealings with patients, colleagues and society. Under this principle, the dentist's primary obligations include dealing with people justly and delivering dental care without prejudice. In its broadest sense, this principle expresses the concept that the dental profession should actively seek allies throughout society on specific activities that will help improve access to care for all.

CODE OF PROFESSIONAL CONDUCT

4.A. Patient Selection

While dentists, in serving the public, may exercise reasonable discretion in selecting patients for their practices, dentists shall not refuse to accept patients into their practice or deny dental service to patients because of the patient's race, creed, color, sex or national origin.

ADVISORY OPINION

4.A.1. Patients with Bloodborne Pathogens

A dentist has the general obligation to provide care to those in need. A decision not to provide treatment to an individual because the individual is infected with Human Immunodeficiency Virus, Hepatitis B Virus, Hepatitis

C Virus or another bloodborne pathogen, based solely on that fact, is unethical. Decisions with regard to the type of dental treatment provided or referrals made or suggested should be made on the same basis as they are made with other patients. As is the case with all patients, the individual dentist should determine if he or she has the need of another's skills, knowledge, equipment or experience. The dentist should also determine, after consultation with the patient's physician, if appropriate, if the patient's health status would be significantly compromised by the provision of dental treatment.

4.B. Emergency Service

Dentists shall be obliged to make reasonable arrangements for the emergency care of their patients of record. Dentists shall be obliged when consulted in an emergency by patients not of record to make reasonable arrangements for emergency care. If treatment is provided, the dentist, upon completion of treatment, is obliged to return the patient to his or her regular dentist unless the patient expressly reveals a different preference.

4.C. Justifiable Criticism

Dentists shall be obliged to report to the appropriate reviewing agency as determined by the local component or constituent society instances of gross or continual faulty treatment by other dentists. Patients should be informed of their present oral health status without disparaging comment about prior services. Dentists issuing a public statement with respect to the profession shall have a reasonable basis to believe that the comments made are true.

ADVISORY OPINION

4.C.1. Meaning of "Justifiable"

Patients are dependent on the expertise of dentists to know their oral health status. Therefore, when informing a patient of the status of his or her oral health, the dentist should exercise care that the comments made are truthful, informed and justifiable. This may involve consultation with the previous treating dentist(s), in accordance with applicable law, to determine under what circumstances and conditions the treatment was performed. A difference of opinion as to preferred treatment should not be communicated to the patient in a manner which would unjustly imply mistreatment. There will necessarily be cases where it will be difficult to determine whether the comments made are justifiable. Therefore, this section is phrased to address the discretion of dentists and advises against unknowing or unjustifiable disparaging statements against another dentist. However, it should be noted that, where comments are made which are not supportable and therefore unjustified, such comments can be the basis for the institution of a disciplinary proceeding against the dentist making such statements.

4.D. Expert Testimony

Dentists may provide expert testimony when that testimony is essential to a just and fair disposition of a judicial or administrative action.

ADVISORY OPINION

4.D.1. Contingent Fees

It is unethical for a dentist to agree to a fee contingent upon the favorable outcome of the litigation in exchange for testifying as a dental expert.

4.E. Rebates and Split Fees

Dentists shall not accept or tender "rebates" or "split fees."

Section 5 Principle: Veracity *("truthfulness")*

The dentist has a duty to communicate truthfully.

> This principle expresses the concept that professionals have a duty to be honest and trust-worthy in their dealings with people. Under this principle, the dentist's primary obligations include respecting the position of trust inherent in the dentist-patient relationship, communicating truthfully and without deception, and maintaining intellectual integrity.

CODE OF PROFESSIONAL CONDUCT

5.A. Representation of Care

Dentists shall not represent the care being rendered to their patients in a false or misleading manner.

From American Dental Association: *American Dental Association principles of ethics and code of professional conduct,* Chicago, 2008, Author. Copyright © 2008 American Dental Association.

ADVISORY OPINIONS

5.A.1. Dental Amalgam and Other Restorative Materials

Based on current scientific data, the ADA has determined that the removal of amalgam restorations from the non-allergic patient for the alleged purpose of removing toxic substances from the body, when such treatment is performed solely at the recommendation or suggestion of the dentist, is improper and unethical. The same principle of veracity applies to the dentist's recommendation concerning the removal of any dental restorative material.

5.A.2. Unsubstantiated Representations

A dentist who represents that dental treatment or diagnostic techniques recommended or performed by the dentist has the capacity to diagnose, cure or alleviate diseases, infections or other conditions, when such representations are not based upon accepted scientific knowledge or research, is acting unethically.

5.B. Representation of Fees

Dentists shall not represent the fees being charged for providing care in a false or misleading manner.

ADVISORY OPINIONS

5.B.1. Waiver of Copayment

A dentist who accepts a third party[1] payment under a copayment plan as payment in full without disclosing to the third party[1] that the patient's payment portion will not be collected, is engaged in overbilling. The essence of this ethical impropriety is deception and misrepresentation; an overbilling dentist makes it appear to the third party[1] that the charge to the patient for services rendered is higher than it actually is.

5.B.2. Overbilling

It is unethical for a dentist to increase a fee to a patient solely because the patient is covered under a dental benefits plan.

5.B.3. Fee Differential

Payments accepted by a dentist under a governmentally funded program, a component or constituent dental society sponsored access program, or a participating agreement entered into under a program of a third party[1] shall not be considered as evidence of overbilling in determining whether a charge to a patient, or to another third party[1] in behalf of a patient not covered under any of the aforecited programs constitutes overbilling under this section of the *Code*.

5.B.4. Treatment Dates

A dentist who submits a claim form to a third party[1] reporting incorrect treatment dates for the purpose of assisting a patient in obtaining benefits under a dental plan, which benefits would otherwise be disallowed, is engaged in making an unethical, false or misleading representation to such third party.[1]

5.B.5. Dental Procedures

A dentist who incorrectly describes on a third party[1] claim form a dental procedure in order to receive a greater payment or reimbursement or incorrectly makes a non-covered procedure appear to be a covered procedure on such a claim form is engaged in making an unethical, false or misleading representation to such third party.[1]

5.B.6. Unnecessary Services

A dentist who recommends and performs unnecessary dental services or procedures is engaged in unethical conduct.

5.C. Disclosure of Conflict of Interest

A dentist who presents educational or scientific information in an article, seminar or other program shall disclose to the readers or participants any monetary or other special interest the dentist may have with a company whose products are promoted or endorsed in the presentation. Disclosure shall be made in any promotional material and in the presentation itself.

5.D. Devices and Therapeutic Methods

Except for formal investigative studies, dentists shall be obliged to prescribe, dispense, or promote only those devices, drugs and other agents whose complete formulae are available to the dental profession. Dentists shall have the further obligation of not holding out as exclusive any device, agent, method or technique if that representation would be false or misleading in any material respect.

ADVISORY OPINIONS

5.D.1. Reporting Adverse Reactions

A dentist who suspects the occurrence of an adverse reaction to a drug or dental device has an obligation to communicate that information to the broader medical and dental community, including, in the case of a serious adverse event, the Food and Drug Administration (FDA).

5.D.2. Marketing or Sale of Products or Procedures

Dentists who, in the regular conduct of their practices, engage in or employ auxiliaries in the marketing or sale of products or procedures to their patients must take care not to exploit the trust inherent in the dentist-patient relationship for their own financial gain. Dentists should not induce their patients to purchase products or undergo procedures by misrepresenting the product's value, the necessity of the procedure or the dentist's professional expertise in recommending the product or procedure.

In the case of a health-related product, it is not enough for the dentist to rely on the manufacturer's or distributor's representations about the product's safety and efficacy. The dentist has an independent obligation to inquire into the truth and accuracy of such claims and verify that they are founded on accepted scientific knowledge or research.

Dentists should disclose to their patients all relevant information the patient needs to make an informed purchase decision, including whether the product is available elsewhere and whether there are any financial incentives for the dentist to recommend the product that would not be evident to the patient.

5.E. Professional Announcement

In order to properly serve the public, dentists should represent themselves in a manner that contributes to the esteem of the profession. Dentists should not misrepresent their training and competence in any way that would be false or misleading in any material respect.[2]

5.F. Advertising

Although any dentist may advertise, no dentist shall advertise or solicit patients in any form of communication in a manner that is false or misleading in any material respect.[2]

ADVISORY OPINIONS

5.F.1. Articles and Newsletters

If a dental health article, message or newsletter is published under a dentist's byline to the public without making truthful disclosure of the source and authorship or is designed to give rise to questionable expectations for the purpose of inducing the public to utilize the services of the sponsoring dentist, the dentist is engaged in making a false or misleading representation to the public in a material respect.[2]

5.F.2. Examples of "False or Misleading"

The following examples are set forth to provide insight into the meaning of the term "false or misleading in a material respect."[2] These examples are not meant to be all-inclusive. Rather, by restating the concept in alternative language and giving general examples, it is hoped that the membership will gain a better understanding of the term. With this in mind, statements shall be avoided which would:

a) contain a material misrepresentation of fact,
b) omit a fact necessary to make the statement considered as a whole not materially misleading,
c) be intended or be likely to create an unjustified expectation about results the dentist can achieve, and
d) contain a material, objective representation, whether express or implied, that the advertised services are superior in quality to those of other dentists, if that representation is not subject to reasonable substantiation.

Subjective statements about the quality of dental services can also raise ethical concerns. In particular, statements of opinion may be misleading if they are not honestly held, if they misrepresent the qualifications of the holder, or the basis of the opinion, or if the patient reasonably interprets them as implied statements of fact. Such statements will be evaluated on a case by case basis, considering how patients are likely to respond to the impression made by the advertisement as a whole. The fundamental issue is whether the advertisement, taken as a whole, is false or misleading in a material respect.[2]

5.F.3. Unearned, Nonhealth Degrees

A dentist may use the title Doctor or Dentist, DDS, DMD or any additional earned, advanced academic degrees in health service areas in an announcement to the public. The announcement of an unearned academic degree may be misleading because of the likelihood that it will indicate to the public the attainment of specialty or diplomate status.

For purposes of this advisory opinion, an unearned academic degree is one which is awarded by an educational institution not accredited by a generally recognized accrediting body or is an honorary degree.

The use of a nonhealth degree in an announcement to the public may be a representation which is misleading because the public is likely to assume that any degree announced is related to the qualifications of the dentist as a practitioner.

Some organizations grant dentists fellowship status as a token of membership in the organization or some other form of voluntary association. The use of such fellowships in advertising to the general public may be misleading because of the likelihood that it will indicate to the public attainment of education or skill in the field of dentistry.

Generally, unearned or nonhealth degrees and fellowships that designate association, rather than attainment, should be limited to scientific papers and curriculum vitae. In all instances, state law should be consulted. In any review by the council of the use of designations in advertising to the public, the council will apply the standard of whether the use of such is false or misleading in a material respect.[2]

5.F.4. Referral Services

There are two basic types of referral services for dental care: not-for-profit and the commercial. The not-for-profit is commonly organized by dental societies or community services. It is open to all qualified practitioners in the area served. A fee is sometimes charged the practitioner to be listed with the service. A fee for such referral services is for the purpose of covering the expenses of the service and has no relation to the number of patients referred. In contrast, some commercial referral services restrict access to the referral service to a limited number of dentists in a particular geographic area. Prospective patients calling the service may be referred to a single subscribing dentist in the geographic area and the respective dentist billed for each patient referred. Commercial referral services often advertise to the public stressing that there is no charge for use of the service and the patient may not be informed of the referral fee paid by the dentist. There is a connotation to such advertisements that the referral that is being made is in the nature of a public service. A dentist is allowed to pay for any advertising permitted by the *Code*, but is generally not permitted to make payments to another person or entity for the referral of a patient for professional services. While the particular facts and circumstances relating to an individual commercial referral service will vary, the council believes that the aspects outlined above for commercial referral services violate the *Code* in that it constitutes advertising which is false or misleading in a material respect and violates the prohibitions in the *Code* against fee splitting.[2]

5.F.5. Infectious Disease Test Results

An advertisement or other communication intended to solicit patients which omits a material fact or facts necessary to put the information conveyed in the advertisement in a proper context can be misleading in a material respect. A dental practice should not seek to attract patients on the basis of partial truths which create a false impression.[2]

For example, an advertisement to the public of HIV negative test results, without conveying additional information that will clarify the scientific significance of this fact, contains a misleading omission. A dentist could satisfy his or her obligation under this advisory opinion to convey additional information by clearly stating in the advertisement or other communication: "This negative HIV test cannot guarantee that I am currently free of HIV."

5.G. Name of Practice

Since the name under which a dentist conducts his or her practice may be a factor in the selection process of the patient, the use of a trade name or an assumed name that is false or misleading in any material respect is unethical. Use of the name of a dentist no longer actively associated with the practice may be continued for a period not to exceed one year.[2]

ADVISORY OPINION

5.G.1. Dentist Leaving Practice

Dentists leaving a practice who authorize continued use of their names should receive competent advice on the legal implications of this action. With permission of a departing dentist, his or her name may be used for more than one year, if, after the one year grace period has expired, prominent notice is provided to the public through such mediums as a sign at the office and a short statement on stationery and business cards that the departing dentist has retired from the practice.

5.H. Announcement of Specialization and Limitation of Practice

This section and Section **5.I** are designed to help the public make an informed selection between the practitioner who has completed an accredited program beyond the dental degree and a practitioner who has not completed such a program. The special areas of dental practice approved by the American Dental Association and the designation for ethical specialty announcement and limitation of practice are: dental public health, endodontics, oral and maxillofacial pathology, oral and maxillofacial radiology, oral and maxillofacial surgery, orthodontics and dentofacial orthopedics, pediatric dentistry, periodontics and prosthodontics. Dentists who choose to announce specialization should use "specialist in" or "practice limited to" and shall limit their practice exclusively to the announced special area(s) of dental practice, provided at the time of the announcement such dentists have met in each approved specialty for which they announce the existing educational requirements and standards set forth by the American Dental Association. Dentists who use their eligibility to announce as specialists to make the public believe that specialty services rendered in the dental office are being rendered by qualified specialists when such is not the case are engaged in unethical conduct. The burden of responsibility is on specialists to avoid any inference that general practitioners who are associated with specialists are qualified to announce themselves as specialists.

GENERAL STANDARDS

The following are included within the standards of the American Dental Association for determining the education, experience and other appropriate requirements for announcing specialization and limitation of practice:

1   The special area(s) of dental practice and an appropriate certifying board must be approved by the American Dental Association.

2   Dentists who announce as specialists must have successfully completed an educational program accredited by the Commission on Dental Accreditation, two or more years in length, as specified by the Council on Dental Education and Licensure, or be diplomates of an American Dental Association recognized certifying board. The scope of the individual specialist's practice shall be governed by the educational standards for the specialty in which the specialist is announcing.

3   The practice carried on by dentists who announce as specialists shall be limited exclusively to the special area(s) of dental practice announced by the dentist.

STANDARDS FOR MULTIPLE-SPECIALTY ANNOUNCEMENTS

The educational criterion for announcement of limitation of practice in additional specialty areas is the successful completion of an advanced educational program accredited by the Commission on Dental Accreditation (or its equivalent if completed prior to 1967)[3] in each area for which the dentist wishes to announce. Dentists who are presently ethically announcing limitation of practice in a specialty area and who wish to announce in an additional specialty area must submit to the appropriate constituent society documentation of successful completion of the requisite education in specialty programs listed by the Council on Dental Education and Licensure or certification as a diplomate in each area for which they wish to announce.

ADVISORY OPINIONS

5.H.1. Dual Degreed Dentists

Nothing in Section 5.H shall be interpreted to prohibit a dual degreed dentist who practices medicine or osteopathy under a valid state license from announcing to the public as a dental specialist provided the dentist meets the educational, experience and other standards set forth in the *Code* for specialty announcement and further providing that the announcement is truthful and not materially misleading.

5.H.2. Specialist Announcement of Credentials in Non-Specialty Interest Areas

A dentist who is qualified to announce specialization under this section may not announce to the public that he or she is certified or a diplomate or otherwise similarly credentialed in an area of dentistry not recognized as a specialty area by the American Dental Association unless:

1 The organization granting the credential grants certification or diplomate status based on the following: a) the dentist's successful completion of a formal, full-time advanced education program (graduate or postgraduate level) of at least 12 months' duration; and b) the dentist's training and experience; and c) successful completion of an oral and written examination based on psychometric principles; and

2 The announcement includes the following language: [Name of announced area of dental practice] is not recognized as a specialty area by the American Dental Association.

Nothing in this advisory opinion affects the right of a properly qualified dentist to announce specialization in an ADA-recognized specialty area(s) as provided for under Section 5.H of this *Code* or the responsibility of such dentist to limit his or her practice exclusively to the special area(s) of dental practice announced. Specialists shall not announce their credentials in a manner that implies specialization in a non-specialty interest area.

5.I. General Practitioner Announcement of Services

General dentists who wish to announce the services available in their practices are permitted to announce the availability of those services so long as they avoid any communications that express or imply specialization. General dentists shall also state that the services are being provided by general dentists. No dentist shall announce available services in any way that would be false or misleading in any material respect.[2]

ADVISORY OPINIONS

5.I.1. General Practitioner Announcement of Credentials in Non-Specialty Interest Areas

A general dentist may not announce to the public that he or she is certified or a diplomate or otherwise similarly credentialed in an area of dentistry not recognized as a specialty area by the American Dental Association unless:

1 The organization granting the credential grants certification or diplomate status based on the following: a) the dentist's successful completion of a formal, full-time advanced education program (graduate or postgraduate level) of at least 12 months' duration; and b) the dentist's training and experience; and c) successful completion of an oral and written examination based on psychometric principles;

2 The dentist discloses that he or she is a general dentist; and

3 The announcement includes the following language: [Name of announced area of dental practice] is not recognized as a specialty area by the American Dental Association.

5.I.2. Credentials in General Dentistry

General dentists may announce fellowships or other credentials earned in the area of general dentistry so long as they avoid any communications that express or imply specialization and the announcement includes the disclaimer that the dentist is a general dentist. The use of abbreviations to designate credentials shall be avoided when such use would lead the reasonable person to believe that the designation represents an academic degree, when such is not the case.

NOTES

1 A third party is any party to a dental prepayment contract that may collect premiums, assume financial risks, pay claims, and/or provide administrative services.

2 Advertising, solicitation of patients or business or other promotional activities by dentists or dental care delivery organizations shall not be considered unethical or improper, except for those promotional activities which are false or misleading in any material respect. Notwithstanding any *ADA Principles of Ethics and Code of Professional Conduct* or other standards of dentist conduct which may be differently worded, this shall be the sole standard for determining the ethical propriety of such promotional activities. Any provision of an ADA constituent or component society's code of ethics or other standard of dentist conduct relating to dentists' or dental care delivery organizations' advertising, solicitation, or other promotional activities which is worded differently from the above standard shall be deemed to be in conflict with the *ADA Principles of Ethics and Code of Professional Conduct.*

3 Completion of three years of advanced training in oral and maxillofacial surgery or two years of advanced training in one of the other recognized dental specialties prior to 1967.

IV. INTERPRETATION AND APPLICATION OF *PRINCIPLES OF ETHICS AND CODE OF PROFESSIONAL CONDUCT*

The foregoing *ADA Principles of Ethics and Code of Professional Conduct* set forth the ethical duties that are binding on members of the American Dental Association. The component and constituent societies may adopt additional requirements or interpretations not in conflict with the *ADA Code*.

Anyone who believes that a member-dentist has acted unethically may bring the matter to the attention of the appropriate constituent (state) or component (local) dental society. Whenever possible, problems involving questions of ethics should be resolved at the state or local level. If a satisfactory resolution cannot be reached, the dental society may decide, after proper investigation, that the matter warrants issuing formal charges and conducting a disciplinary hearing pursuant to the procedures set forth in the ADA *Bylaws*, Chapter XII. PRINCIPLES OF ETHICS AND CODE OF PROFESSIONAL CONDUCT AND JUDICIAL PROCEDURE. The Council on Ethics, Bylaws and Judicial Affairs reminds constituent and component societies that before a dentist can be found to have breached any ethical obligation the dentist is entitled to a fair hearing.

A member who is found guilty of unethical conduct proscribed by the *ADA Code* or code of ethics of the constituent or component society, may be placed under a sentence of censure or suspension or may be expelled from membership in the Association. A member under a sentence of censure, suspension or expulsion has the right to appeal the decision to his or her constituent society and the ADA Council on Ethics, Bylaws and Judicial Affairs, as provided in Chapter XII of the ADA *Bylaws*.

INDEX

Advisory opinions are designated by their relevant section in parentheses, e.g. (2.D.1.)

Bibliography and Suggested Readings

Adler MJ: *Aristotle for everybody*, Toronto, 1978, Bantam Books.

American Association of Dental Schools: Curriculum guidelines in dental professional ethics, *J Dent Educ* 53:144, 1989.

American Dental Association Council on Ethics, Bylaws and Judicial Affairs: *ADA principles of ethics and code of professional conduct*, Chicago, 2008, American Dental Association.

American Dental Hygienists' Association: *Code of ethics for dental hygienists*, Chicago, 1998-1999, Author.

Anderson RM, Davidson PL, Atchison KA, et al: Pipeline, profession, and practice program: evaluating change in dental education, *J Dent Educ* 69(2):239, 2005.

Angeles PA: *Dictionary of philosophy*, New York, 1981, Harper & Row.

Barish NH, Barish AM: The ethical dilemma of the dental hygienist, *J Am Coll Dent* 39:169, 1972.

Beauchamp TL, Childress JF: *Principles of biomedical ethics*, ed 4, New York, 1994, Oxford University Press.

Bebeau MJ: Teaching ethics in dentistry, *J Dent Educ* 49:236, 1985.

Bebeau MJ, Born DO, Ozar DT: The development of a professional role orientation inventory, *J Am Coll Dent* 60(2):27, 1993.

Bebeau MJ, Thoma SJ: The impact of a dental ethics curriculum on moral reasoning, *J Dent Educ* 58(9):684, 1994.

Bebeau MJ, Rest JR, Narváez DF: Beyond the promise: a perspective for research in moral education, *Educ Res* 28(4):18, 1999.

Bebeau MJ, Kahn J: *Ethical issues in community dental health*. In Gluck GM, Morganstein WM, eds: Jong's community dental health, ed 5, St Louis, 2002, Mosby, pp 425-445.

Beemsterboer PL: Competency in allied dental education, *J Dent Educ* 11:19, 1994.

Beemsterboer PL: Developing an ethic of access to care in dentistry, *J Dent Educ* 70(11):212, 2006.

Beemsterboer PL, Odom JG, Pate TD, et al: Issues of academic integrity in U.S. dental schools, *J Dent Educ* 64:833, 2000.

Beemsterboer PL, Odom J: Ethical principles in clinical decision making, *Calif Dent Hyg J* 17(1): 7-9, 12, 2001.

Benjamin M, Curtis J: *Ethics in Nursing*, ed 2, New York, 1986, Oxford University Press.

Biddington WR: The dental policy perspective, *J Am Coll Dent* 57:20, 1990.

Biddington WR, Nash DA: A person within a community of persons, *J Am Coll Dent* 51:12, 1984.

Black's law dictionary, ed 8, St Paul, MN, 2004, West Publishing Company.

Brennan M, Oliver R, Harvey B, et al: *Ethics and law for the dental team*, United Kingdom, 2006, PasTest Ltd.

Chambers DW: Toward a competency-based curriculum, *J Dent Educ* 57:790, 1993.

Chambers DW: The professions, *J Am Coll Dent* 71(4):57, 2004.

Chambers DW: Access denied: invalid password, *J Dent Educ* 70(11):1146, 2006.

Chambers DW: Basic oral health needs: a public priority, *J Dent Educ* 70(11):1159, 2006.

Chambers DW: Moral communities, *J Dent Educ* 70(11):1226, 2006.

Chi MT, Glaser R, Farr M: *The nature of expertise*, Hillsdale, NJ, 1988, Lawrence Erlbaum.

Childress JF: *Who should decide? Paternalism in health care*, New York, 1982, Oxford University Press.

Cianflone D, Riccelli AE: Ethical considerations for dental hygienists in private practice settings, *J Dent Hyg* 65:277, 1991.

Corsino BV, Patthoff DE: The ethical and practical aspects of acceptance and universal patient acceptance, *J Dent Educ* 70(11):1198, 2006.

Crall JJ: Access to oral health care: professional and societal considerations, *J Dent Educ* 70(11):1133, 2006.

Davidson JA: *Legal and ethical considerations for dental hygienists and assistants*, St Louis, 2000, Mosby.

DePaola DP: Beyond the university: leadership for the common good. In *75th anniversary summit conference discussion papers and proceedings*, American Association of Dental Schools, Washington, DC October 12-13, 1998.

Dharamsi S: Building moral communities? First, do no harm, *J Dent Educ* 70(11):1235, 2006.

Dharamsi S, MacEntee M: Dentistry and distributive justice, *Soc Sci Med* 55:323, 2002.

Dreyfus HL, Dreyfus SE: *Mind over machine*, New York, 1986, The Free Press.

Edelstein BL: Disparities in oral health and access to care: findings of national surveys, *Ambulatory Pediatr* 2(suppl 2):141, 2002.

Edge RS, Groves JR: *Ethics of health care: a guide for clinical practice,* ed 2, Albany, NY, 1999, Delmar.

Francoeur RT: *Biomedical ethics: a guide to decision making,* New York, 1983, John Wiley & Sons.

Garcia RI: Addressing oral health disparities in diverse populations, *J Am Dent Assoc* 136:1210, 2005.

Garetto LP, Yoder KM: Basic oral health needs: a professional priority? *J Dent Educ* 70(11):1166, 2006.

Gilligan C: *In a different voice,* Cambridge, MA, 1982, Harvard University Press.

Haden NK, Catalanotto FA, Alexander CJ, et al: Improving the oral health status of all Americans: roles and responsibilities of academic dental institutions: the report of the ADEA president's commission, *J Dent Educ* 67:563, 2003.

Hall MA, Ellman IM: *Health care law and ethics,* St. Paul, MN, 1990, West Publishing Company.

Jones LB: Professionalism and ethics, *J Am Dent Assoc* 57:40, 1990.

Jonsen AR, Siegler M, Winslade WJ: *Clinical ethics: a practical approach to ethical decisions in clinical medicine,* ed 5, New York, 2002, McGraw-Hill.

Josephson M: *Making ethical decisions,* ed 3, Marina del Rey, CA, 1995, Josephson Institute of Ethics.

Kenny N, Shelton W: *Lost virtue: professional character development in medical education,* United Kingdom, 2006, Emerald Group Publishing Ltd.

Kimbrough VJ, Lautar CJ: *Ethics, jurisprudence, and practice management in dental hygiene,* Englewood Cliffs, NJ, 2003, Prentice Hall.

Kohlberg L: Stage and sequence: The cognitive development approach to socialization. In Goslin D, ed: *Handbook of socialization theory and research,* Chicago, 1969, Rand McNally, pp 347-480.

Kohlberg L: The cognitive-developmental approach to moral education. In Scharf P, ed: *Readings in moral education,* Minneapolis, MN, 1978, Winston Press.

Krepp GL: *Effective communication in multicultural health care settings,* Thousand Oaks, CA, 1994, Sage Publications.

Loewy EH: *Textbook of healthcare ethics,* ed 2, New York, 1996, Plenum Press.

Lustbader W: *Counting on kindness,* New York, 1991, The Free Press.

McNally M: Rights access and justice in oral health care, *J Am Coll Dent* 70:56, 2003.

Minton AJ, Shipka TA: *Philosophy: paradox & discover,* ed 2, New York, 1982, McGraw-Hill.

Morris WO: *The dentist's legal advisor,* Philadelphia, 1995, CV Mosby.

Motley WE: *Ethics, jurisprudence and history for the dental hygienist,* ed 3, Philadelphia, 1983, Lea & Febiger.

Motley WE: *History of the American Dental Hygienists' Association,* Chicago, 1986, American Dental Hygienists' Association.

Nash DA: Ethics in dentistry: review and critique of *Principles of Ethics and Code of Professional Conduct, J Am Dent Assoc* 109:597, 1984.

Nash DA: Ethics. . .and the quest for excellence in the profession, *J Dent Educ* 49:229, 1985.

Nash PJ, Nash DA, Hutton JL: Moral reasoning and clinical performance of student dentists, *J Dent Educ* 46:721, 1982.

Newell KJ, Young LJ, Yamoor CM: Moral reasoning in dental hygiene students, *J Dent Educ* 49:79, 1985.

Noddings N: *Caring: a feminine approach to ethics and moral education,* Berkeley, 1994, University of California Press.

Nordstom NK, Soller H, Odom JG: Hygiene practice ethics, *Can Dent Assoc J* 16:27, 1988.

Odom JG: Formal ethics instruction in dental education, *J Dent Educ* 46:553, 1982.

Odom JG: Parameters and goals for teaching ethics, *Ohio Dent J* 58:36, 1984.

Odom JG: Recognizing and resolving ethical dilemmas in dentistry, *Med Law* 4:543, 1985.

Odom JG: The status of dental ethics instruction, *J Dent Educ* 52:306, 1988.

O'Toole B: Promoting access to oral health care: more than professional ethics is needed, *J Dent Educ* 70(11):1217, 2006.

Ozar DT: Three models of professionalism and professional obligation in dentistry, *J Am Dent Assoc* 110(2):173, 1985.

Ozar DT: Applying systems thinking to oral health care: commentary on Dr. Patricia H. Werhane's article, *J Dent Educ* 70(11):1196, 2006.

Ozar DT: Ethics, access, and care, *J Dent Educ* 70(11):1139, 2006.

Ozar DT, Sokol DJ: *Dental ethics at chairside: professional principles and practical applications,* ed 2, Washington, DC, 2002, Georgetown University Press.

Pathoff DE: How did we get here? Where are we going? Hopes and gaps in access to oral health care, *J Dent Educ* 70(11):1125, 2006.

Peltier B: Codes and colleagues: is there support for universal patient acceptance? *J Dent Educ* 70(11):1221, 2006.

Pollack BR: *Risk management in dental practice in community dental health,* ed 3, St Louis, 1993, CV Mosby.

Pritchard MS: Professional integrity: thinking ethically, Lawrence, KS, 2006, University of Kansas Press.

Purtilo RB: *Ethical dimensions in the health professions,* ed 2, Philadelphia, 1993, WB Saunders.

Purtilo R, Haddad A: *Health professional and patient interaction,* ed 7, Philadelphia, 2007, Saunders Elsevier.

Reich W, ed: *Encyclopedia of bioethics,* ed 2, New York, 1992, The Free Press.

Rule JT, Veatch RM: *Ethical questions in dentistry,* Chicago, 1993, Quintessence.

Rule JT, Veatch RM: *Ethical questions in dentistry,* ed 2, Chicago, 2004, Quintessence.

Smith DH: Band-Aid solutions to problems of access: their origins and limits, *J Dent Educ* 70(11):1170, 2006.

Stern DT: *Measuring medical professionalism,* New York, 2006, Oxford University Press.

Sullivan WM: *Work and integrity,* ed 2, San Francisco, 2005, Jossey-Bass.

Thiroux JP: *Ethics: theory and practice,* New York, 1986, Macmillan.

Tong R: *Feminist approaches to bioethics,* Oxford, United Kingdom, 1997, Westview Press.

U.S. Department of Health and Human Services: *A plan to eliminate craniofacial, oral and dental health disparities,* Rockville, MD, 2002, National Institutes of Health.

U.S. Department of Health and Human Services: *Healthy people 2010: understanding and improving health,* ed 2, Rockville, MD, 2000, National Institutes of Health.

U.S. Department of Health and Human Services: *Oral health in America: a report of the surgeon general,* Rockville, MD, 2000, National Institutes of Health.

Vaughn, LD, Harvey L: The team approach to risk management, *Access* May-June:42, 2008.

Veatch RM: *A theory of medical ethics,* New York, 1981, Basic Books.

Veatch RM: *Medical ethics,* Boston, 1989, Jones & Bartlett.

Welie JVM: Is dentistry a profession? Part I: professionalism defined, *J Can Dent Assoc* 70(8):529, 2004.

Welie JVM: Is dentistry a profession? Part II: hallmarks of professionalism, *J Can Dent Assoc* 70(9):599, 2004.

Welie JVM: Is dentistry a profession? Part III: future challenges, *J Can Dent Assoc* 70(10):675, 2004.

Welie JVM: *Justice in oral health care: ethical and educational perspectives,* Milwaukee, WI, 2006, Marquette University Press.

Weinstein BD: *Dental ethics,* Philadelphia, 1993, Lea & Febiger.

Werhane PH: Access, responsibility, and funding: a systems thinking approach to universal access to oral health, *J Dent Educ* 70(11):1184, 2006.

Williams JR: *Dental ethics manual,* Ferney-Voltaire, France, 2007, FDI World Dental Federation.

Woodall IR: *Leadership, management and role delineation,* St Louis, 1977, CV Mosby.

Glossary

abandonment   discontinuation of a patient/provider relationship once it has been established

accreditation   a nongovernmental process for ensuring that a predetermined set of standards has been met; used to assure the public that the graduates of a particular program are prepared to practice

allegation   an assertion, claim, or statement of an individual in a legal proceeding

amoral   to be without morals; that which is indifferent to morality

autonomous   independent and self-determining

autonomy   the principle of self-determination in a person; the right to participate in and decide on a course of action without undue influence; provides the foundation for a right to privacy and the ability to choose

battery   the commission of bodily harm against another person

beneficence   the principle of promoting good or well-being

breach of contract   the act of breaking a contract, agreement, promise, or legal duty by failing to perform a promised or required act

character   collectively, the qualities that define a person or group of persons; a person's moral nature

civil action   legal action taken to protect the private rights of individuals

civil law   legal matters other than criminal ones; includes torts and contractual agreements

civil rights   the rights granted residents of the United States by the Constitution and legislative acts passed after the Civil War; freedom of speech, the right to vote, and freedom from discrimination

code of ethics   a set of rules or guidelines that address the ethical standards of a professional group

competency   having the knowledge, skill, and ability to perform a prescribed set of tasks or duties independently and with confidence

confidentiality   that which is entrusted or held in secret; the precept by which information shared by a patient during the course of receiving health care is kept in confidence by the health care provider

consequentialism   the theory that the rightness or wrongness of actions is determined by consequences; also called *teleology*

contributory negligence   an action or lack of action that contributes to the harm or injury of an individual and negatively affects his or her health status

criminal action   a legal action taken in a court of law to protect society

criminal law   a body of laws established for the purpose of preventing harm to society; describes what conduct is criminal and prescribes the punishment for criminal conduct; may be codified into criminal or penal codes

defamation   the act of maliciously making a false statement that injures another's reputation; termed *libel* if a written statement, *slander* if an oral statement

defendant   a person being sued in a civil case or charged with a crime

dental record   a written comprehensive, ongoing file of assessment findings, treatments rendered, notations, and contacts with the dental patient

deposition   a discovery method, out of court, in which information is given under oath of testimony of a party or witness and recorded by a court reporter; can be subject to cross-examination

discovery   the process by which or period during which each party involved in a lawsuit obtains information concerning the facts of the lawsuit; includes depositions, interrogations, and record copying

discrimination   the act of treating persons differently based on factors they cannot control, such as age, handicapping condition, race, or gender

distributive justice   the just allocation and distribution of resources for the good of society

due process   the right of fair application of laws or regulations for each person; a process established to ensure fairness and equity

duty   action or conduct based on moral or legal obligation

emancipated minor   an individual younger than 18 years who is independent of a parent; laws can vary from state to state

employment   a situation in which an individual works for payment

Equal Employment Opportunity Commission   the federal agency that investigates claims of employment discrimination and sexual harassment

ethical analysis   the process by which ethical decisions are made using a structured format

ethical dilemma   a situation in which two or more ethical principles are in conflict

ethical theory   a systematic examination of morals involving critical reflection and analysis about what is right and wrong

ethics the inquiry into the nature of morality or moral acts; values by which human beings live in relation to other human beings, nature, a higher power, and/or themselves

federal laws laws enacted and upheld by the U.S. government

fiduciary relationship a relationship based on responsibility between the patient and the health care provider

harassment the act of annoying or threatening a person by word or deed

Hippocratic oath an oath, written by a physician in the fourth century, that is the foundation for most ethical codes in health care

impaired professional an individual who has undergone professional training but who is no longer able to function in a professional capacity because of illness or substance abuse

implied not specifically stated or written but capable of being inferred by action(s)

incident reporting a written report that details the aspects of an accident or unusual situation

informed consent the act of providing information to and ensuring the understanding of a patient regarding treatment risks, treatment options, and the nature of the disease or problem

injury any wrong or damage done to another person, his or her rights, reputation, or property

injury causation the required link between a patient's injury and a dental hygienist's breach of duty (i.e., the patient's injury must be caused by the dental hygienist's breach of duty)

intentional tort a civil wrong that occurs when an individual intends the results of an action

justice the principle that deals with fairness and the allocation of what people earn or deserve

licensure a process regulated by a governmental agency in which individuals are authorized to perform certain functions

malpractice professional services, such as performed by a dentist or dental hygienist, done without reasonable care or skill or in violation of ethics

moral dilemma situation in which obligations and responsibilities are in conflict

moral distress frustration from perceived powerlessness when what is happening appears to be wrong and the person is unable to act ethically

morality that which is right and good; the quality of an action with regard to right and wrong

moral principle a mode of choosing that which is universal

moral reasoning the formulation of a morally ideal course of action; the process of judging what one ought to do in a specific situation

moral sensitivity   the process of interpreting a situation from a moral perspective; involves making inferences about thoughts, feelings, and perceptions of others; understanding

moral uncertainty   a state of questioning whether a moral obligation exists and/or the scope of that obligation

moral weakness   a state in which moral responsibilities and personal inclinations are in conflict

negligence   a lack of reasonable and prudent care resulting in harm

nonconsequentialism   theory where an action is right when it conforms to a duty or rule; also called deontological ethics or Kantian ethics

nonmaleficence   the principle that states the duty to avoid harming the patient, summarized in the phrase "do no harm"

oath   a solemn promise to do something or to follow some guideline(s)

obligation   a duty to conform to a rule or custom

paternalism   an act or action based on doing good for a patient, in the manner that a father would, but that is done without the patient's full knowledge; an approach that limits a patient's autonomy

peer review   the process of allowing professional colleagues to critically examine treatment provided in a dental or dental hygiene case and render an opinion on the appropriateness of that treatment

prima facie duty   considering only one single moral principle, the first principle to act on over another equally compelling principle; the duty that may be primary

primum non nocere   a Latin term meaning "first, do no harm"

professional autonomy   the concept that a professional who provides care for a patient, thereby establishing a provider-patient relationship, is not obligated to provide that care if it would involve performing unethical services

professional code   the written standards that detail the responsibilities of a particular group

professionalism   the quality of performing with the skill, knowledge, and abilities of a professional person; the possession of specialized knowledge and skill in a field of human endeavor

professional traits   characteristics desirable in a health care professional

quality assessment   a process used systematically and continuously to assess the quality of the patient care delivery system for the purpose of improvement

quality improvement   system to collect information that will lead to the improvement of procedures, processes, and outcomes

quid pro quo   a Latin term meaning "something for something"

regulation   a rule or restriction

relativism   the theory that truth is not absolute but is relative to circumstances, individual beliefs, cultural background, or other factors

risk factors   listing of structures, procedures, or processes that could lead to undesired outcomes

sanction   a penalty attached to a law to gain compliance

scope of practice   the broad range of duties legally defined for a particular health care provider

sexual harassment   a form of discrimination; involves unwelcome talk or touching or other actions regarding sexual activity

standard   a quality or specific level of performance

standard of care   the level and quality of care expected of a reasonable and prudent practitioner

statute of limitations   the state law or part of a specific statute that specifies the period during which legal action must be taken

statutory law   a body of law created by acts of the legislature

supervision   the act of directing or observing the activities of another person

tort   a civil wrong in which another's person or property is harmed as a result of negligent or intentional acts

trait   a characteristic

unintentional tort   a civil wrong that occurs when an individual does not intend the results of an action

utilitarianism   the theory that an action is right when it conforms to a rule of conduct or judgment providing the greatest balance of good or evil; also termed *deontology*

value   a principle or concept considered worthwhile

veracity   truth-telling; honesty

virtue ethics   a theory that focuses on the character traits of an individual rather than on the individual's specific behavior

Index

Page numbers followed by *f* Indicates figures; *t*, tables; *b* boxes.